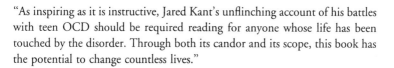

"As inspiring as it is instructive, Jared Kant's unflinching account of his battles with teen OCD should be required reading for anyone whose life has been touched by the disorder. Through both its candor and its scope, this book has the potential to change countless lives."

—Jeff Bell, author of Rewind Replay, Repeat:
A Memoir of Obsessive-Compulsive Disorder

"What a remarkable book! Jared Kant and his co-authors have produced a revealing, first-hand look at OCD that manages to be brutally honest, yet at the same time tremendously supportive and reassuring. I admire Jared's bravery and his willingness to let the world see his descent into this terrible illness as well as his eventual recovery. Young people with OCD will find the insights in this book to be informative, frightening, humorous, and hopeful–sometimes all at once. If you are a teenager or young adult with OCD, this book is a must-read."

*—David F. Tolin, Ph.D., Director, Anxiety Disorders Center,
The Institute of Living; Adjunct Associate Professor,
Yale University School of Medicine, and author of* Buried in
Treasures: Help for Compulsive Acquiring, Saving, and Hoarding

"*The Thought That Counts* is *The Catcher in the Rye* for adolescents and young adults with OCD. It tells the reader's story as well as the author's. After reading this book, the OCD sufferer is no longer alone and has information about ways to manage his or her OCD."

*—Patricia B. Perkins, J.D., former Executive
Director of the OC Foundation*

"Finally, an articulate and intelligent OCD book for teens that tells it as only someone who has been there and back can tell it. It is a much-needed addition that fills a gap in the ever-growing body of OCD resources for those who suffer from this life-disrupting problem. It is a practical combination of a well-written narrative of one young person's struggle to find himself and establish a meaningful life in the face of a serious mental illness, together with accurate and professionally guided information."

—Fred Penzel, Ph.D., author of Obsessive-Compulsive Disorders:
A Complete Guide to Getting Well and Staying Well

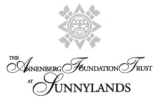

THE
ANNENBERG FOUNDATION TRUST
AT SUNNYLANDS

The Annenberg Foundation Trust at Sunnylands'
Adolescent Mental Health Initiative

Patrick E. Jamieson, Ph.D., *series editor*

Other books in the series
For young people

*Mind Race: A Firsthand Account of One Teenager's Experience
With Bipolar Disorder*
Patrick E. Jamieson, Ph.D., with Moira A. Rynn, M.D.

*Monochrome Days: A Firsthand Account of One Teenager's
Experience With Depression*
Cait Irwin, with Dwight L. Evans, M.D., and Linda Wasmer Andrews

*What You Must Think of Me: A Firsthand Account of One
Teenager's Experience With Social Anxiety Disorder*
Emily Ford, with Michael Liebowitz, M.D., and Linda Wasmer Andrews

*Next to Nothing: A Firsthand Account of One Teenager's Experience
With an Eating Disorder*
Carrie Arnold, with B. Timothy Walsh, M.D.

*Me, Myself, and Them: A Firsthand Account of One Young Person's
Experience With Schizophrenia*
Kurt Snyder, with Raquel E. Gur, M.D., Ph.D., and Linda Wasmer Andrews

*Chasing the High: A Firsthand Account of One Young Person's Experience With
Substance Abuse*
Kyle Keegan, with Howard B. Moss, M.D. (forthcoming, 2008)

Eight Stories Up: An Adolescent Chooses Hope Over Suicide
DeQuincy A. Lezine, Ph.D., with David Brent, M.D. (forthcoming, 2008)

For parents and other adults

If Your Adolescent Has Depression or Bipolar Disorder
Dwight L. Evans, M.D., and Linda Wasmer Andrews

If Your Adolescent Has an Eating Disorder
B. Timothy Walsh, M.D., and V. L. Cameron

If Your Adolescent Has an Anxiety Disorder
Edna B. Foa, Ph.D., and Linda Wasmer Andrews

If Your Adolescent Has Schizophrenia
Raquel E. Gur, M.D., Ph.D., and Ann Braden Johnson, Ph.D.

The Thought That Counts

A Firsthand Account of One Teenager's Experience With Obsessive-Compulsive Disorder

Jared Douglas Kant

with Martin Franklin, Ph.D., and Linda Wasmer Andrews

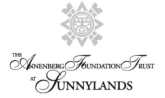

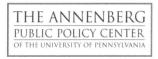

The Annenberg Foundation Trust at Sunnylands'
Adolescent Mental Health Initiative

THE ANNENBERG
PUBLIC POLICY CENTER
OF THE UNIVERSITY OF PENNSYLVANIA

OXFORD
UNIVERSITY PRESS

2008

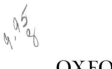

OXFORD
UNIVERSITY PRESS

Oxford University Press, Inc., publishes works that further
Oxford University's objective of excellence
in research, scholarship, and education.

The Annenberg Foundation Trust at Sunnylands
The Annenberg Public Policy Center of the University of Pennsylvania
Oxford University Press

Oxford   New York
Auckland   Cape Town   Dar es Salaam   Hong Kong   Karachi
Kuala Lumpur   Madrid   Melbourne   Mexico City   Nairobi
New Delhi   Shanghai   Taipei   Toronto

With offices in
Argentina   Austria   Brazil   Chile   Czech Republic   France   Greece
Guatemala   Hungary   Italy   Japan   Poland   Portugal   Singapore
South Korea   Switzerland   Thailand   Turkey   Ukraine   Vietnam

Published by Oxford University Press, Inc.
198 Madison Avenue, New York, New York 10016

www.oup.com

Library of Congress Cataloging-in-Publication Data

Kant, Jared (Jared Douglas)
The thought that counts : a firsthand account of one teenager's experience with obsessive-
compulsive disorder / by Jared Kant with Martin Franklin, and Linda Wasmer Andrews.
    p. cm. — (The Annenberg Foundation Trust at Sunnylands' adolescent mental health
initiative)
"The Annenberg Public Policy Center of the University of Pennsylvania."
Includes bibliographical references and index.
ISBN 978-0-19-531688-9 (cloth) — ISBN 978-0-19-531689-6 (pbk)
1. Kant, Jared (Jared Douglas)—Health.   2. Obsessive-compulsive disorder in
adolescence—Patients—United States.   I. Franklin, Martin, 1963–   II. Andrews, Linda
Wasmer.   III. Annenberg Public Policy Center.   IV. Title.
RJ506.O25K36 2008
616.85'22700835—dc22
[B]   2007035115

9 8 7 6 5 4 3

Printed in the United States of America
on acid-free paper

Contents

Foreword

The Adolescent Mental Health Initiative (AMHI) was created by The Annenberg Foundation Trust at Sunnylands to share with mental health professionals, parents, and adolescents the advances in treatment and prevention now available to adolescents with mental health disorders. The Initiative was made possible by the generosity and vision of Ambassadors Walter and Leonore Annenberg, and the project was administered through the Annenberg Public Policy Center of the University of Pennsylvania in partnership with Oxford University Press.

The Initiative began in 2003 with the convening, in Philadelphia and New York, of seven scholarly commissions made up of over 150 leading psychiatrists and psychologists from around the country. Chaired by Drs. Edna B. Foa, Dwight L. Evans, B. Timothy Walsh, Martin E. P. Seligman, Raquel E. Gur, Charles P. O'Brien, and Herbert Hendin, these commissions were tasked with assessing the state of scientific research on the prevalent mental disorders whose onset occurs predominantly between the ages of 10 and 22. Their collective findings now appear in a book for mental health professionals and policy makers titled *Treating and Preventing Adolescent Mental Health Disorders* (2005). As the first product of the Initiative, that book also identified a research agenda that would best advance our ability to prevent and treat these disorders, among them anxiety disorders, depression and bipolar disorder, eating disorders, substance abuse, and schizophrenia.

The second prong of the Initiative's three-part effort is a series of smaller books for general readers. Some of the books are designed primarily for parents of adolescents with a specific mental health disorder. And some, including this one, are aimed at adolescents themselves who are struggling with a mental illness. All of the books draw their scientific information in part from the AMHI professional volume, presenting it in a manner that is accessible to general readers of different ages. The "teen books" also feature the real-life story of one young person who has struggled with—and now manages—a given mental illness. They serve as both a source of solid research about the illness and as a roadmap to recovery for afflicted young people. Thus they offer a unique combination of medical science and firsthand practical wisdom in an effort to inspire adolescents to take an active role in their own recovery.

The third part of the Sunnylands Adolescent Mental Health Initiative consists of two Web sites. The first, www.CopeCareDeal.org, addresses teens. The second, www.oup.com/us/teenmentalhealth, provides updates to the medical community on matters discussed in *Treating and Preventing Adolescent Mental Health Disorders,* the AMHI professional book.

We hope that you find this volume, as one of the fruits of the Initiative, to be helpful and enlightening.

Patrick Jamieson, Ph.D., *Series Editor*
Adolescent Risk Communication Institute
Annenberg Public Policy Center
University of Pennsylvania
Philadelphia, PA

Preface

I was 12 years old when I came to terms with the idea that I would live my life with obsessive-compulsive disorder (OCD). I distinctly remember looking up at the sky and saying, "All right, fine, but something good better come out of this." Strangely enough, I remember thinking to myself at the time that, if I ever found my way out of the fog, I would like to write a book about my experiences.

Eleven years later, Sarah Harrington, an associate editor from Oxford University Press, called the Obsessive-Compulsive Foundation in New Haven, Connecticut, looking for the author of some articles I had written for the organization. Patricia Perkins, the foundation's executive director, called my house, and a book was born. Today, after a year of writing and rewriting and writing some more, I finally have reached the culmination of what is almost a lifelong goal.

With this book, I hope to bring meaning to chaos, to bring order to disorder—no pun intended. As someone who has battled OCD for more than half his life, I feel a great affinity with those of you who are facing the same battle. I empathize with your struggles, because they are my struggles, too.

I won't lie to you: It's not easy being a teenager or young adult with OCD. In fact, it can be a terrifyingly wild ride at first, before you find the right treatment for you. It is my sincere hope as both a writer and a comrade in the fight against mental illness that you will find direction and solace in these pages.

Faces Behind the Pages

This book is, first and foremost, a memoir of my journey through adolescent OCD. It wasn't a smooth ride, and in the chapters to come, you'll feel every jarring bump in the road and see every looming obstacle. But before we look back, let's see where my travels have brought me so far.

Managing OCD at school was a particular challenge for me. Yet in 2006, I graduated at the top of my college class with a bachelor's degree in English and creative writing. After graduation, I began writing this book. And soon after that, while I was still working on the manuscript, I landed a job as a clinical research assistant in the Body Dysmorphic Disorder Clinic at Massachusetts General Hospital, one of the premier hospitals in the country. As you'll learn in Chapter 5, body dysmorphic disorder (BDD) is a disorder that often goes hand in hand with OCD, so my job has been a nice complement to my writing.

To ensure that the clinical and scientific parts of this book are accurate, I have been lucky enough to team up with one of the nation's foremost authorities on OCD. Martin E. Franklin, Ph.D., is an associate professor of clinical psychology and psychiatry, as well as clinical director of the Center for the Treatment and Study of Anxiety at the University of Pennsylvania School of Medicine. At the center, Dr. Franklin's work has focused primarily on the development and evaluation of OCD treatments. Previously, Dr. Franklin was co-investigator and clinical supervisor on research funded by the National Institute of Mental Health (NIMH) that looked at both pediatric and adult OCD. Currently, he is principal investigator on another NIMH-funded study looking at the effectiveness of adding cognitive-behavioral therapy to the treatment of OCD in children and teens who have already shown partial improvement with medication.

All told, Dr. Franklin has spent decades studying OCD and treating hundreds of people with this often disabling condition. By weaving together his professional expertise with my personal experiences, this book helps you look at OCD from every angle.

The third member of our writing team is Linda Wasmer Andrews, a journalist who has specialized in mental health topics since the early 1980s. Together, my coauthors and I have created a unique book that combines deeply personal insights with the most up-to-date scientific information. It's my story, but it's your story, too. With that in mind, we've also provided practical tips and useful resources for coping with OCD.

How to Use This Book

Each chapter of this book opens with a section titled "My Story." This is where I recount my journey through OCD. Sometimes it was harrowing, sometimes it was humorous— but it was always real. The second half of each chapter is titled "The Big Picture," and that's where we provide a broader context for my individual experiences. It's in this section that you'll find the essential facts you need to give your own OCD story a happy ending.

The people, places, and events described in my memoir are true. Pseudonyms have been used to protect the privacy of individuals. But otherwise, I've tried to provide an honest, un-varnished account of what I went through and how I felt at the time.

In the years since my diagnosis, public attitudes toward OCD have changed dramatically. It doesn't have the same sticky, id-iosyncratic connation that it once had. Instead, it's regarded now with curiosity and interest. Although negative stereotypes are still prevalent, there is also greater acceptance and under-standing of OCD as a biological disease that responds to proven treatments.

It is my greatest hope as a writer and a person with OCD that those of us with this disorder will learn to not only move past our disease, but also move forward with our lives. We can support each other along the way and shirk off the stigma that surrounds mental illness to this day. Together, we can make each other stronger.

The Thought That Counts

Chapter One

On Second (and Third and Fourth) Thought: Obsessions and Compulsions

My Story

When I was much younger, long before the symptoms manifested, I was a happy kid. At least, most of my memories from being younger seem to center around a knowledge that I was somehow special.

I was one of those kids who would study an anthill instead of playing soccer. Rather than longing for the prefabricated action figures and toys that were advertised on television, I would construct cities out of building blocks. I could be entertained for whole days this way. As I got older, the things I built began to reflect the trouble that was to come. Like a horse that can smell rain, I could smell the storm.

Overall, though, I was a gentle kid. I loved to read; I was reading at a twelfth-grade level in first grade. I would sit around the house, looking at the various accoutrements of modern living, furiously studying how they worked. I was computer literate in kindergarten.

Looking back on it, I had the whole world, so to speak, in my hands. I grew up in an affluent community with a loving, hard-working family. My mother taught the third grade and my father was an attorney. I used to sit in his office while he was at meetings, sifting through the contents of his drawers and building small vehicles out of binder clips and paperclips, pens and pencils.

To this day, people at my father's work talk about the time I turned a box of red coffee stirrers and a few staples into a convincing-looking lobster sculpture. Suffice to say, I was a creative kid, but I didn't worry about impressing anyone. It's peculiar to think that, when I was much younger, I was confident that people would like me just by virtue of the fact that I was, well, me. It's sad how in our culture that sort of self-esteem through innocence is incinerated by the fifth grade.

I realize now that I had some peculiarities, but they didn't seem to cause much of a problem. I was useless at team sports, but I could hold my own in any discussion. I grew up with the same cultural influences and the same, or at least similar, musical tastes as any young boy. I listened to pretty much everything.

My family traveled. My sister and I passionately hated each other while remaining inseparable best friends, and my dad was my hero. I went through all the various "when I grow up" stages as other kids. I wanted to be a policeman-plumber-carpenter-doctor with a high-profile position in the government, defending the country.

Essentially, aside from being a horribly picky eater, overly shy, and constantly mindful of a desire to remain clean at all times, I was a normal kid. I suppose they really mean it when they say puberty changes everything.

Diseases, Physical and Mental

When I was about 11, there was a big scare in Africa regarding the Ebola virus. This deadly plague was particularly gruesome because it caused blood to leak under the skin and seep from body orifices. The virus made headlines day after day in the national media. It seemed that everyone was talking about the possibility of Ebola spreading to the United States and the potential hazard it might pose.

Being scientifically minded, I decided to read up on everything related to the Ebola virus. I sought out documents from the Centers for Disease Control and Prevention in Atlanta, and I read them all carefully, with attention to every detail. What I didn't notice until too late was that my fascination with Ebola stemmed from an uneasy feeling that I could somehow become exposed to the virus simply by reading about it. Jackets of books about the subject, illustrated with brightly colored images of cells infected with the disease, were taboo. I was afraid to touch them for fear that the disease would somehow be transmitted through the images.

In retrospect, I can see other early warning signs as well. When I would walk into my middle school, I invariably would enter from a certain angle. The building was designed by someone who was obviously more interested in form than function, and it was hard to navigate. I would start in the foyer and suddenly find myself in the locker room, without a hint as to how I got there.

I started always leaving the building by the same route I had used entering it. That is, if I went down a certain set of corridors, through certain doors, and into certain classrooms, then when I exited, I had to take that same route to get outside. When I was lazy and failed to do this, I would feel a tremendous sense of discomfort, an uneasiness in my stomach.

Around this time, I also began to wash my hands more thoroughly. The soap had to be antibacterial, and I would only wipe my hands on fresh towels. Sometimes I would just get up from class and go wash my hands, using the bathroom as an excuse.

The truth is, I was obsessing long before I was diagnosed with obsessive-compulsive disorder (OCD).

At the time, I wasn't actively aware of what I was doing. Today, though, I can see the seeds of illness in these behaviors. The truth is, I was obsessing long before I was diagnosed with obsessive-compulsive disorder (OCD).

Disasters Waiting to Happen

In addition to disease, disaster became my other obsession. On the Internet, I would watch footage of the bombing of Hiroshima over and over. At first, I thought that it was amazing. And it was. The atomic bomb changed the world, although not for the better. It let humans know that our destructive capabilities were far beyond what we had ever anticipated. All of this was racing through my mind. I was convinced that if I wasn't careful, I would somehow trigger a cataclysmic world war that would end life as we knew it. I marveled at how other people could be so oblivious to the potential disasters that were springing up all around us.

When I began to get acne, my anxiety intensified. One day I was scrubbing my face. I looked in the mirror, and wouldn't you know it, there were spots on me. They were slightly raised, a little red, with white in the middle. The skin around these areas was irritated, tender to the touch, and I was terrified. I ran into my mother and father's room, sure that I had contracted a dread disease. I could feel it in me. I had the sensation of being infected without actually having so much as a cold. My father turned on the lamp, looked at the rash, and told me it was pimples.

I began using the library computers to look up online articles about all the diseases that can cause skin bumps. There is, for the record, a vast number of such diseases, and I was overwhelmed by an inordinate amount of information. Eventually, I started to believe that I was getting skin cancer. I had read in a magazine that prolonged exposure to the sun could lead to skin cancer, and this fact took on a life of its own in my mind.

Walking through the halls of the school became more and more of a task as time went on. I began having acute anxiety over the idea of going the wrong way. I was afraid of all sorts of things, but I suppressed my fears because I thought they were stupid. They still scared me, though, and the more I suppressed them, the more powerful the fears became. When it was time for me to go to summer camp, I had already figured out that something was not right.

Less-Than-Happy Camper

The summer when I was 11 years old was a turning point in my life. When I got on the bus to go away to camp that year, I felt a new and intense anxiety that reached beyond homesickness or second-guessing.

I was confused. I had attended the same camp a year earlier, and it was easily one of the best experiences of my young life. I had learned to kayak, sail, hike, shoot, and build a fire. I met friends that lasted years afterward.

This time at camp was different, though. Within a few weeks, maybe a month, I had stopped leaving the cabin. Most people thought I was trying to get out of mandatory exercise and were irritated that I got away with it. Then a counselor came into the cabin and found me sobbing and listening to my Walkman, headphones loud, with my butt sticking in the air, rocking back and forth. This counselor and I had gotten to know each other the year before, and in choking gasps, I cried out for him to sit with me.

A week later, I was on a bus trip, surrounded by children sucking on obscenely sweet, giant balls of candy. Every time I looked down at mine or at a friend's, I felt the overwhelming urge to vomit, for this was a lollipop you could use more than once. Some of them had softer shells from the saliva of their owners. The butterscotch smell was overwhelming. I saw germs and diseases, infections and all manner of ills where the other kids saw a sugary treat.

As the bus ride continued, I began to think about an escape I had become fixated on, something to do with space aliens. I think, looking back, that I secretly hoped the aliens would take me away and make me better. I clung desperately to that idea.

Within days, I became convinced that I was actually one of the aliens. I looked at the pictures of my cat, my sister, and my mother and father, and I prayed for their forgiveness when they discovered that I was not the boy they believed me to be. Somewhere along the way, I truly lost myself. I knew with frightening certainty that I was not like everyone else.

Invasion of the Mind Snatchers

Around this time, I began to recognize that some of my thoughts seemed wrong. A part of me believed that the only aliens were these thoughts inside my head. Instead of being an intruder, it was I who had been intruded upon. However, another part of me believed that the aliens had planted this doubt in my mind as a fail-safe mechanism to insure that I was a good spy. I was torn between my allegiances. There was that which I wanted to believe, and that which I couldn't help believing. I doubted everything, and it made me get sicker and sicker.

Yet providence was on my side in one respect. Miraculously and mercifully, by sheer chance or divine intervention, a pediatric psychologist had married into the family that owned the camp I was attending. He was alerted about my condition by the counselor who had found me rocking that day.

The psychologist asked questions that seemed to read my mind. I didn't feel distrustful, but I doubted that he could help me. That is, until he told me that there was a name for what was wrong and that thousands of children like me had these kinds of thoughts. Suddenly, it seemed at least possible that I was going to get help.

... he told me that there was a name for what was wrong and that thousands of children like me had these kinds of thoughts.

I still can remember riding home from camp in the family station wagon. The only thing I knew for certain was that I was going on another trip. On some level, I knew I was headed home, but I wasn't quite sure where that was. Still, landmarks along the drive kept poking out at me, prompting me to remember where I had come from.

Writing about it now, I have a profound urge to tear this page out of the notebook, to try and forget what the ride was like. That is exactly why I'm writing this book. For all the pain and tears, the yelling and screaming, the anger and isolation, I'm proud of where I come from. When I say this, mind you, I'm not talking about a small suburb outside of Boston, which is where I grew up. No, I'm talking about the bizarre and often painful past that I first had to endure before I could enjoy the life I have now.

When I spent my first night at my parent's house, home from summer camp, I was absolutely terrified. For while I was sure that things would only get better, I knew, or rather felt, that I was doing something wrong. I had this nagging doubt about everything I did, and it followed me everywhere. This, I would eventually come to know was the disease.

Those first days back home were spent refamiliarizing myself with the objects and obstacles that I had known so well. It was both frightening and embarrassing. The anxiety meant that even tying my own shoes was hard. Taking a shower was an undertaking of epic proportions, and just eating dinner was a battle. I had become the prisoner of an illness that held my mind in an iron grip. The struggle to free myself would last through my teens and into my college years.

The Big Picture

When I was younger, the word "obsession" made me think of infatuation. If a boy fell head over heels for a girl, spending an extraordinary amount of time and energy daydreaming about her and hanging on her every word, people would say, "He's obsessed with that girl." Naturally, it didn't occur to me to use the same word to describe the peculiar thoughts I was having. But as I later realized, there's a big difference between the everyday meaning of obsession and the scientific definition.

In scientific terms, an obsession is a recurring thought or mental image that seems intrusive and inappropriate, and that causes anxiety and distress. It's different from simply being preoccupied with a cute classmate or a favorite hobby, because even after obsessive thoughts start causing serious problems, the person feels powerless to stop thinking them. At some point, the person realizes that the thoughts are controlling him or her instead of the other way around.

Obsessive thoughts aren't just exaggerated worries about real-life concerns. Instead, they're overblown fears and anxieties with little basis in reality. Yet once these thoughts push their way into someone's mind, they refuse to leave no matter how hard the person tries to push them out.

Consider my obsession with images of disease, for instance. Flipping through magazines as a boy, I sometimes came across disturbing images of plague and pestilence, such as flies buzzing over open sores. When I saw such pictures, I carefully avoided touching them. Occasionally, though, I would make a mistake. My finger would drag across the ink on the page until it hit one of the infected people. Whenever this happened, I screamed inside. I ran to the bathroom, slathered myself in soap, and turned the hot water up to boil. I was steaming, and I must have looked like a lobster by the time I emerged from the bathroom.

My reaction to touching the images illustrates another critical point: Obsessive thoughts lead to intense anxiety about something bad or harmful that the person fears will occur. The anxiety is so strong that the person feels compelled to do something—*anything*—to get relief and ward off the feared consequence. That's how compulsions, such as my excessive hand-washing, are born. From a scientific standpoint, then, a compulsion is a repeated act, either behavioral or mental, that a person feels driven to perform in response to an obsession, to keep something bad from happening or to reduce the associated distress.

So What Exactly Is OCD?

As the name implies, OCD is a mental disorder characterized by recurring, uncontrollable obsessions and compulsions. When professionals classify mental illnesses, OCD is lumped together with conditions such as phobias and panic attacks in a category called anxiety disorders. Such disorders involve excessive fear or worry that lasts a long time or keeps coming back. The symptoms cause distress or interfere with the person's usual activities and social relationships.

Of course, everyone worries from time to time. For most people, though, the worries change along with whatever is going on in the person's life at that moment. Obsessions, on the other hand, are more enduring. The same unwanted thoughts keep repeating themselves over and over. Although the exact nature of the thoughts varies from person to person, obsessions often involve concerns about being diseased, dirty, or sinful. Each time the thoughts return, they stir up feelings of fear, distress, disgust, or shame all over again.

When people repeatedly try to neutralize these thoughts or images with another thought, image, or action, a compulsion results. Compulsions often involve rigid routines and rituals that seem nonsensical to outside observers. But to the person with OCD, they have a purpose, because they counteract the anxiety that comes from obsessive thoughts. The problem is that they're only a temporary solution. The thoughts soon come back, and so does the desperate need for relief.

... the more you command yourself not to have an obsessive thought, the stronger and more intense it tends to become.

It's a vicious cycle that is very difficult to break through sheer force of will. In fact, the more you command yourself not to have an obsessive thought, the stronger and more intense it tends to become. Fortunately, there are effective treatments that can help you break free of the cycle and take charge of your life again. These treatments are described in detail in Chapter 4.

VIOLENT OBSESSIONS

Some of the most disturbing obsessions involve violent thoughts and images. People with OCD live in terror that they'll act on these thoughts, which they find abhorrent. However, for those whose violent thoughts truly are due to OCD and not to some other problem, that fear is unfounded. The violent thoughts, like other obsessions, lead to compulsive rituals, not to acts of violence.

Yet the thoughts alone are distressing enough, like having a horror movie playing in your head that you can't turn off. In my case, just at the age when I was approaching sexual awareness, I started to have horrifying visions of myself committing sexual assaults on girls I found attractive. To me, rape is one of the worst things that a person can do to another human being, so I was extremely shaken by these thoughts. Finding relief from such disturbing thoughts and images is one of the most important reasons for seeking professional help.

What Forms Can the Disorder Take?

OCD rituals and routines are the outward signs of inward turmoil. The specific compulsions are as widely varied as the individuals who have them. Yet compulsions tend to fall into general patterns, and professionals use these patterns to classify subtypes of the disorder. Below are seven common subtypes. Keep in mind, though, that many people with OCD develop more than one kind of compulsion.

- Washing and cleaning—This is the most common compulsive behavior in teens. It springs from obsessive thoughts about contamination by germs, poisons, or bodily secretions. To counter such concerns, some people wash their hands excessively—often to the point where their hands become dry, red, and chapped from the constant scrubbing. Others clean their rooms for hours or develop complicated rituals for showering. These same teens may go to great lengths to avoid contamination, such as repeatedly wiping off doorknobs that might be germ-laden or avoiding any object that has touched the floor.

- Checking—People with checking compulsions are consumed by anxiety about potential calamities. To quell their fears, they repeatedly check to make sure the calamity hasn't occurred yet. For instance, students who obsess about losing their homework or textbooks may check again and again to see whether these items are in their backpacks. Of course, it's not unusual to double-check whether you have all your belongings. But those with OCD can become stuck for hours in a fruitless cycle of worrying and checking, worrying and checking.

- Repeating—Like checkers, repeaters often are obsessed with potential disasters. The difference is that the protective rituals they develop have no logical connection to the feared event. For instance, let's say a teenager is wracked with worry about a burglar breaking into the house at night while everyone is asleep. A checker might check over and over to see whether the doors and windows are locked—a logical, if excessive, response to the anxiety. A repeater, on the other hand, might pace for hours around her room following the same path each time—an illogical, yet still excessive, way of warding off burglary. Another group of repeaters say that they repeat actions—for instance, walking up and down the stairs—because the failure to do so would cause unre-

OCD or Quirky Habit?

"Step on a crack, break your mother's back." Stepping over cracks in the sidewalk is a ritual that doesn't have any logical relationship to keeping Mom safe, yet many people still do it. Does this mean they all have the repeating form of OCD? No. Most of us have a few quirky habits or superstitious behaviors. Many people also develop healthy, soothing rituals, such as always reading right before bedtime. There's nothing abnormal about these behaviors so long as they don't cause serious problems. In contrast, OCD rituals consume an inordinate of time and lead to substantial distress or interfere with the ability to get along in daily life.

mitting distress. In these cases, there is no identified feared consequence other than distress. Yet the prospect of not repeating the action to neutralize the distress still seems overwhelming.

- Ordering and arranging—Orderers and arrangers are plagued by worries that something in their environment is not just right. This subtype of compulsion is unusual in that there typically aren't any feared consequences. Instead, there is just a sense of uneasiness that lasts until everything is back in its proper place. To reduce the uneasiness, people with this type of OCD may spend considerable time ordering, arranging, and straightening objects. They often become very upset when their possessions are moved.

- Hoarding—People who compulsively hoard things are driven by constant anxiety about not having what they'll need in the future. Some actively collect items that others would consider useless or excessive. Others simply avoid ever throwing anything away. So while a typical teen

---

Compulsion or Tic?

A student touches every object on her desk in rapid succession, then does it again and again. She wishes she could stop, but she can't seem to control what she's doing. Does she have an ordering compulsion? Maybe. However, it's also possible that she might have a complex tic. Tics are sudden, rapid, repetitive movements or vocalizations that serve no useful purpose. But more complex tics, which involve coordinated patterns of movement in several muscle groups, sometimes look as if they might be purposeful even though they aren't. Examples include touching or tapping objects, hopping, bending, twisting, or outbursts of words or phrases.

Even for the pros, it can be hard to tell the difference between OCD and a complex tic. The task is made more difficult by the fact that many people have both—up to 30% of people with OCD report having had tics at some point in their lives. As a general rule, though, compulsions are preceded by a mental event, such as an obsession or perhaps a feeling of anxiety. Tics, on the other hand, are preceded by a sense of physical tension that builds up until the need for release is almost irresistible, much like the tension before a sneeze. Many compulsive rituals also are more elaborate than even the most complex tics.

---

might want to collect every CD by their favorite bands, a hoarder might collect four copies of each CD or also hang onto the bags and receipts they came with.

- Counting and other mental rituals—Like other people with OCD, those who fall into this category engage in compulsive rituals. The difference is that they perform their rituals entirely within their minds. Examples include counting to oneself, making mental lists, or silently repeating certain words or phrases. Some mental rituals go along with ones that are acted out. For instance, a student who compulsively checks the contents of his backpack might form a mental image of himself going through the pack and confirming that everything is there. Then instead of actually checking the pack again, he can replay the image in his mind. But whether the ritual is done mentally or physically, the purpose is the same: to relieve anxiety and restore a sense of security, if only temporarily.

Life by the Numbers

I felt the tickle in my throat like something had found its way into my esophagus and wanted out. Then my arms began to tingle like an itch that couldn't be scratched. I was in the lobby of the junior high school I had attended for a year. Students congregated there to gossip, talk about their plans for the weekend, and compare notes on which teachers were the hardest. But my mind was preoccupied with something else that day. I was getting more and more antsy that I was going to burst into noise. I became afraid that if I didn't make the sound, if I didn't let the creature inside me go, I would die. The longer I resisted and the more I thought about it, the more I became powerless to resist.

My vocal chords tightened. I felt my jaw clench, and, although most people don't even know we have two sets of vocal cords, I really felt as if mine were becoming asynchronous. Terrified of both this new sensation and what people would think if I let out a loud wail to clear my throat, I tightened my throat to make the sound as quiet as possible.

The sound came out like a frog croaking in a low octave, quick and forced. Some people turned their heads, but they seemed to lose interest very quickly. Then, suddenly, horrified, my attention came to my obsession with numbers. My first experience with tics—sudden, brief, explosive movements or vocalizations—and now I was going to have to tic twice more. That made three. Three is a holy number so I moved to five. My throat started to hurt; I felt like I had bronchitis.

At this point, people were asking me what was wrong. I was reassuring them when, mid-sentence, another one of the buggers seized control and escaped. Three of my friends watched, their eyes

(*continued*)

widening. I had slipped into six, which is like sixty-six, which was my sister's favorite number, which led to the most unholy number, six hundred sixty-six. I had to force another croak out to get to the Lord's number seven. I coughed to cover the sound. Eight was a comfort number, so I tic-coughed again. Thirteen more vocalizations later, I was at twenty one, my voice box screaming in pain. A crowd had gathered around by this point.

When I regained my composure, I suddenly realized that my legs were crossed wrong. Numbers sorted through my head. I settled on five. I crossed and uncrossed my legs once, twice, three times. I was holding myself up with my arms, hands palm downward in an awkward arch. Four. I pushed for five. I thought at this point everyone was judging me. I wanted a paper bag to put over my head, or a curtain to hide behind while my stupid brain sorted out my stupid obsessions so the people in front of me wouldn't have to see any more compulsions. I felt naked.

Then my friend Jessica came over and saved my dying social life. Jessica had a gorgeous smile with a personality and body to match. The whole school loved her. What most people didn't know was that Jessica also had OCD with a side order of Tourette's syndrome, a disorder characterized by frequent physical and vocal tics. Jessica was a master at camouflaging her symptoms. At school, she clapped her hands under the desk, but by using only one hand at a time like a clamshell snapping shut, she minimized the noise. She also licked her lips frequently, but by applying fresh lip gloss afterward, she simply seemed like a connoisseur of lip care products.

We moved down the hall, away from the other students. Then I collapsed, crying softly, and Jessica cradled me. My friend Brad, who was the size of a house but all muscle and heart, stood guard as my own personal bouncer. I was safe and saved. Brad offered to fetch me something, although he admitted he didn't know what could possibly help. I dried my eyes and asked for a glass of water. Then I started to laugh gently in Jessica's arms. Life is essentially ridiculous, but at least for the time being, the balance had been restored.

These days, I just pardon myself and let the noises quietly escape, then get back to whatever I was doing. Unfortunately, there are some people who will make fun of you or judge you because of their own insecurities or just plain cruelty. That's fine. Remember that the unkind behavior of others says more about them than it does about you. And it's more than canceled out by the kindness of true friends.

- Praying and scrupulosity—Scrupulosity refers to an excessive concern about offending God, committing a sin, having blasphemous thoughts, or doing something immoral. There's often a fine line between scrupulosity, on one hand, and being devoutly religious or having a highly developed conscience, on the other. However, the harshly self-critical beliefs of someone with scrupulosity often exceed both religious doctrine and secular law. To make up for perceived wrongdoings, the person may pray compulsively, make the sign of the cross repeatedly, or develop other personal rituals of atonement.

In addition to developing rituals to neutralize their obsessions, people with OCD often start avoiding the things and events that set off their anxiety. For instance, a student with scrupulosity might believe she's cheating if her eyes merely graze the test of a nearby classmate, even if she doesn't look at the answers. To reduce her sense of anxious guilt, the student might silently say a prayer, repeating it to herself so many times that she fails to finish the test. Later this same student might become so worried about cheating that she starts to avoid taking tests, staying home on days when tests are scheduled even when she knows the material.

How Common Is OCD?

OCD can lead to some very strange-looking behavior. One person taps his glass three times before every drink. Another pauses awkwardly during conversations, because she's repeating everything the other person says backward in her mind. And still another repeatedly dresses and undresses, believing this will keep loved ones safe. It might seem that an illness this individualistic would be rare. Yet OCD is more common than you might think. If you notice some OCD-like thoughts and behaviors in yourself, it's good to know that you're not alone.

Full-blown OCD affects about 2.2 million Americans age 18 and older in any given year.

Full-blown OCD affects about 2.2 million Americans age 18 and older in any given year. Studies suggest that up to 1% of younger people may have the disorder as well. Before puberty, the disorder is more common in boys than girls. After puberty, though, girls catch up, and the prevalence of OCD in adolescents and adults is about equal between the sexes.

One-third of adults with the disorder first developed symptoms during childhood. In most other cases, the first symptoms appeared during the teen or young adult years. The obsessions and compulsions usually take hold gradually, although occasionally the onset of problems is more sudden.

What Causes the Disorder?

OCD has long fascinated scientists because it's such a dramatic disease. Past theories blamed it on everything from overly strict toilet training to a faulty moral upbringing. Yet try as they might, researchers failed to find evidence that child-rearing practices or learned attitudes actually cause the disorder. The verdict: Your parents may have punished you for getting dirty or taught you that certain thoughts were bad, but that in itself doesn't mean you'll develop OCD.

Today the main focus has shifted from emotional explanations to genetic and biological ones. There is now a large and growing body of research linking OCD to a malfunctioning brain. Of course, once the disease has taken root, social and environmental factors still may affect how the symptoms are experienced. Stressful situations, for example, may make symptoms worse.

Below is a brief rundown of some factors that may cause or contribute to OCD. Keep in mind that it's a complex disorder, so it may have multiple causes that interact with each other in complicated ways.

BIOLOGICAL FACTORS

OCD seems to be related to changes in the brain's natural chemistry. Neurotransmitters are chemicals that act as messengers within the brain. One such chemical messenger that has been implicated in OCD is serotonin, a neurotransmitter that helps regulate mood, sleep, appetite, and sexual drive. Low levels of serotonin have been linked to both anxiety and depression.

Brain imaging studies have shown that people with OCD tend to have different patterns of brain activity from those seen in either healthy individuals or people with other mental disorders. In particular, the brains of people with OCD often have abnormalities in the circuits that link the orbital cortex, located at the front of the brain, and the basal ganglia, located deeper inside. Serotonin plays an important role in communication between these structures.

However, the strongest evidence linking serotonin to OCD comes from drug treatment studies. Research shows that people with OCD often improve when they take selective serotonin reuptake inhibitors (SSRIs), medications that increase the available supply of serotonin in the brain. As a result, SSRIs are now frequently prescribed along with psychotherapy for treating OCD.

Genetic Factors

Genes also seem to play a key role in OCD. If you have a parent or another close relative with the disorder, your own risk of developing it is increased. The risk is especially high if you have a parent who developed OCD as a child or if you have several relatives with the disorder. You might think that the tendency for OCD to run in families could be explained by children imitating the compulsive behaviors they see their parents perform. However, research has shown that, when both a parent and a child have OCD, they usually don't have the same symptoms. For instance, a parent who is a compulsive checker might raise a child who is a compulsive washer. This bolsters the argument that heredity rather than learning is at play.

Recently, scientists at the National Institutes of Health (NIH) discovered that a certain genetic variation is about twice as common in people with OCD as in those without the disorder. The variation occurs in the serotonin transporter (SERT) gene, which helps regulate serotonin concentrations in the brain and is a major site of action for SSRI medications. Yet inheriting the SERT variation isn't enough to produce OCD by itself, according to the NIH researchers. Instead, it may simply make a person more vulnerable to developing the disorder when other contributing factors also are present.

Environmental Factors

While OCD has its roots in biology and genetics, people with the disorder, like everybody else, also are affected by what's happening in the world around them. In some people with OCD, stressful life events may worsen the intrusive thoughts and compulsive rituals that are hallmarks of the disorder. In my case, I was already showing subtle signs of OCD before

I went to camp that summer when I was 11. But the stress of going away to camp made my symptoms much worse, to the point where I attracted professional attention for the first time.

Interactions with other people don't cause OCD, but they may make the disorder worse once it's present. Some relationships are very stressful. In other cases, family and friends may inadvertently strengthen compulsive rituals by going along with them, no matter how irrational or inconvenient the rituals might be. Often the loved ones have the best of intentions, only wanting to keep the peace or temporarily make the sick person feel better. In the long run, though, family and friends who are too cooperative with OCD may wind up making it stronger.

> *In the long run, family and friends who are too cooperative with OCD may wind up making it stronger.*

THE INFECTION CONNECTION

One more strange-but-true fact about OCD: In a very small number of children, OCD or tics start suddenly and dramatically after a strep throat. Tics are sudden, repetitive, purposeless movements or vocalizations, such as eye blinking, facial grimacing, shoulder shrugging, head jerking, throat clearing, sniffing, or grunting. The catchy name for this uncommon form of childhood OCD is PANDAS (short for pediatric autoimmune neuropsychiatric disorders associated with streptococcal infections).

To be diagnosed with PANDAS, a child must have OCD or a tic disorder that began between age three and puberty. Over time, the symptoms also must show a pattern of dramatic ups and downs. They start abruptly, then slowly improve. But if the child catches another strep infection, the symptoms abruptly worsen again. Along with obsessions, compulsions, and/or tics, children with PANDAS often have other symptoms, such as hyperactivity, trouble concentrating, irritability, sadness, sleep problems, bedwetting, joint pains, and anxiety about separating from their parents.

Recent research has helped clarify how strep might trigger OCD. The immune system is a network of cells, tissues, and organs that defend the body against attacks by foreign invaders, such as bacteria or viruses. When the immune system encounters something foreign in the body, it makes antibodies, molecules designed to destroy or inactivate that invader. In the case of PANDAS, this process goes awry. Antibodies meant to attack strep bacteria mistakenly act on a certain brain enzyme. This disrupts communication between brain cells, which is thought to cause the OCD symptoms or tics.

By definition, PANDAS is a childhood illness. As more research is done, it's always possible scientists might discover that some teens and adults have immune-mediated OCD as well. For now, though, it's only known to occur in children—and not in very many children, at that. Just because you've had strep throat in the past and have OCD now doesn't mean it's a case of PANDAS. In fact, almost all school-age children catch strep throat at some point, but very few get OCD as a result. PANDAS is only considered as a possible diagnosis when there's an extremely close relationship between a strep infection and the start or worsening of OCD or tics.

Keep in mind that OCD itself is not contagious—a key fact that some people misunderstand. At one point after it became public knowledge that I had OCD, several classmates told me they were concerned about contracting the disorder from me. At the time, I felt like a leper, suddenly outcast to the desert, only to be visited by the strong-willed and the merciful. Today, though, I recognize this type of uninformed statement as a chance to gently educate other people about my illness. Nothing dispels a baseless fear or negative stereotype like the truth.

Fitting In

In junior high school, it's sometimes literally impossible to not feel that you are being judged or that someone is making fun of you. As a conspicuous hand washer and someone who frequented his adviser's office more than usual, I was automatically suspect. The more I attempted to pass their scrutiny off as if nothing was wrong, the more obvious it became to me that other people were judging me—or at least, that was my perception of the situation.

When I would go to the cafeteria, if I could be so persuaded, I had to have the hottest possible plates, which were, as a matter of fact, too hot to handle without getting burned. I knew that other people had previously eaten off the same plates, and I was willing to endure a little burning to reduce my risk of contamination. At some point, I also started to sterilize the silverware with a small cigarette lighter under the table. Every time someone saw this, I felt a rush of blood to my head and wanted to become invisible.

One day, someone made a joke about the size of the lockers and dared me to squeeze into mine, so I did. Much to my amazement, it was a good fit, and after that, the locker became my personal refuge. I went there to hide, to count, to cry alone—in short, to do whatever it was that other people didn't need to see. Before long, hiding in my locker had become a compulsive ritual. I felt that I had to spend a certain amount of time in the locker every day, and that it was imperative that I open the locker door just right.

As you can probably guess, the day finally came when I was observed by a group of people as I emerged from my hiding spot. This was worse than being caught repeatedly tapping my foot in the doorway of the classroom. It was worse than coming to the class with red, scalded hands. It was even worse than having toilet paper on my shoe or my fly unzipped. After all, wouldn't *you* have a hard time not formulating an opinion about a kid who apparently lived in his locker?

(continued)

In an effort to save face, I pointed out that it took great skill to contort myself into the shape of a pile of books. Then I accused onlookers of being jealous that they, too, couldn't hide out in their lockers until the bell rang. Sweat was dripping from my armpits. I thought briefly that my odds of finding a girlfriend had just plummeted to near zero. I felt, in a word, destitute.

To my surprise, a popular kid in the class thought this was the coolest thing he had ever seen. Most people just skipped class by traveling the halls. I actually had a place to hang out and listen to music. I gained a reputation as something of a contortionist, and I ran with it. It was a whole lot better than being an outcast. Was I embarrassed? Absolutely. But in retrospect, I think this was one of the more amusing things I ever did in school.

What's the Least I Need to Know?

Having OCD is no picnic. The unwanted thoughts and ritualistic behaviors can take over your life and make it nearly impossible to do the other things you want to do. You may realize that your constant washing or counting or checking doesn't make sense, but you still feel powerless to stop—and you probably hate the feeling of being so out of control.

If you're like me, you may find it a relief to finally put a name to the problem. OCD is a real and serious illness, not some figment of your imagination or sign of a character flaw. It's a biologically based disease, and you can't just talk yourself out of it any more than you could talk yourself out of having diabetes or asthma. The

... with proper treatment and hard work, you can learn to let go of your obsessions and gain control over your compulsions.

good news is that, like these other diseases, OCD can be treated. And with proper treatment and hard work, you can learn to let go of your obsessions and gain control over your compulsions. It won't be easy, but I'm living proof that it's possible to fight back against OCD and win.

Chapter Two

Slippery Slope to the Hospital: Diagnosis and Hospitalization

My Story

The first thing I learned about psychiatrists is that they have candy. At least, that was true of the psychiatrist I saw after returning home from summer camp. He seemed to understand that something sweet was needed to counter the bitter feelings and experiences we were about to explore.

This psychiatrist formally diagnosed my OCD when I was 11. The shock of what that diagnosis meant came in stages. Ironically, my initial reaction was to feel overjoyed. I was happy and grateful to know that there was a name for what I was going through. It wasn't until later that the gravity of the situation sank in.

Then the anger took over. I didn't want to talk it out, but I did want to yell. One of the first things the psychiatrist taught me was that, in the proper setting, yelling is just fine. It wasn't my fault that I had this disease. I hadn't done anything to deserve it, and it was, simply put, unfair. It was okay and even natural to be angry, but I needed to learn how to harness that energy and use it for something constructive.

That was the long-term goal. In the short term, I did a lot of screaming, a lot of kicking, and a lot of running. I wore myself out crying. I hit the couch with my fists. It took a long time to learn how to use my anger to propel myself through the impediments that stood in the way of getting better.

I learned very quickly that having OCD was not like breaking an arm. As a young, affluent American, I was used to a quick fix. I thought that OCD was like a really bad headache; I would take some magic pill, and it would go away. I was considerably disappointed to learn that it wouldn't be nearly as simple as that.

> *I thought that OCD was like a really bad headache; I would take some magic pill, and it would go away.*

Darkness Falls Early

There I was, not yet a teenager, and I was being told that I had to cope with a serious illness. I didn't want to cope. Instead, I wanted to set fire to myself and run down the street. I asked the sky to strike me with lightning. I wanted the whole world to know that I refused to accept the burden that had just been given to me.

The depression that followed hit hard and fast. The sky became less blue, the light grew dimmer. Almost overnight, my world began to darken, and hope seemed to wither. My eating habits turned from poor to wretched, and I forgot how to talk to people. For me, it seemed there was no solace.

Around this time, my taste in music turned dark as well. I was introduced by my friends to bands such as Nine Inch Nails, Marilyn Manson, and Rage Against the Machine. When you're young and something as monstrously unfair as OCD falls in your lap, hearing adults tear into lyrics about injustice and shred away on guitars is vindication in its purest form. I became addicted, and to this day, I still listen to music by these bands. It reminds me that I'm not alone.

By sixth grade, I was skipping lunch to listen to another favorite band, Cannibal Corpse. The fast, furious, rhythmic pounding of the bass ripped into me, and while the music played, I allowed myself to be at peace with the war inside my head. Unfortunately, when the music ended, I faced a real world that seemed more ominous and hopeless than I could have imagined before.

I grew up fast. I grew up young. I saw life as vastly unforgiving. Anger was a constant, and depression earmarked my days. It was during this period that I saw my dad cry for the first time. I think watching me suffer broke my dad's heart. But eventually, his heart healed and grew stronger than ever.

Meanwhile, almost overnight, my mom amassed a seemingly endless supply of books about OCD. Even though she was emotionally drained and probably terrified, she still had an intellectual hunger for information that would help her and my dad understand their son.

Around this time, the Obsessive-Compulsive Foundation hosted a conference in Boston. My mom attended, and it was there that she first learned about the dedicated group of people whose goal and purpose was to inform the public about this potentially debilitating disease. At the conference, my mom gathered an armful of helpful literature about every facet of the illness. In the wake of devastation, she brought home a small bag of hope.

The World Gets Scarier

Puberty was difficult enough, but puberty with OCD verged on ludicrous. When I first reintroduced myself to society after learning of my diagnosis, I felt as if everyone was leering at me, aware that something was wrong. I could feel their eyes burning into me, but I couldn't communicate what was going on.

The world was a scary place, and things that had produced mild anxiety when I was well were absolutely terrifying now. The division between what was actually an illness-related train of thought and what was a natural, albeit exaggerated, concern blurred to the point of obscurity. Everything became a matter of avoidance. I couldn't go into a public bathroom alone. I couldn't tie my shoes, take a walk, or even draw on a piece of paper without becoming terrified. The anxiety built up to such an extreme that I lost my appetite completely. My mom and dad would encourage me to eat at dinnertime, but I couldn't.

Douglas Adams, one of my favorite authors, suggested that the most terrifying and cruel thing you could do was to show a person exactly where in the universe he or she was. In his famous novel *The Hitchhiker's Guide to the Galaxy*, Adams explored the idea of this awareness as a form of torture. The way it worked was to show someone a map displaying the infinite complexity and enormity of the universe, with a sign pointing to that person's exact place in it. The theory was that nothing could be more traumatic than the comparison of one's minuscule place within all that vastness.

When I first read the section of the novel that explains this theory, I burst out laughing. Adams was a man who got it. There really was nothing more terrifying than knowing how small I was in this bizarre and often cruel world.

Toxic Fears and Poisonous Thoughts

I remember one night when my mom called me downstairs to help prepare the salad for dinner. She wanted to get me out of my bedroom, where I was ruminating on matters that were screaming through my head. When I reached the kitchen, my mom handed me the paring knife, and we started to work on getting each vegetable cut up and cleanly dumped into the bowl.

As soon as I felt the rush of blood to my face, I knew what it meant: An obsession was soon to follow, and sure enough, it did. This particular intrusive thought was a horrific one, the type of harming fear that was becoming my dominant obsession. In my head, I visualized myself poisoning the salad dressing. It was nothing more than a flicker of an image—quick, brutal, and to the point.

In my head, I visualized myself poisoning the salad dressing.

Everyone has this sort of disturbing thought from time to time. In fact, when surveyed, over 90% of people without OCD indicated as much, and the rest were probably lying. However, the thought is usually dismissed immediately—so quickly that it doesn't even register with most people. For people with OCD, though, the thought can linger, and that's what happened to me.

I put the knife down on the cutting board and walked away from the counter. My mom looked up in time to see my eyes widen in fear and beads of sweat form on my brow. This reaction had become all too familiar to her, and she gave my dad a wordless look that spoke volumes about her concern.

My mom was the first to ask what was wrong. I told my parents that I didn't know how or why the salad might have been poisoned, but I felt it was important to inform them that they shouldn't eat the salad or anything that had come in contact with the salad or the dressing. I was uncertain where this notion came from or what my motive could possibly have been for poisoning the salad. As I later learned, the lack of any reasonable explanation for a fear was one clue that it might be an obsession. Yet no matter how absurd the notion of poisoning seemed, it was still terrifying, and I urged my parents to throw out the salad.

My dad—rather bravely, I thought—said that they would take their chances. He pointed out that it was extremely unlikely that I had found a way to slip arsenic or cyanide into the salad without having access to such poisons or a reason to use them. This made me feel better for half a second, and then I grew more concerned. I realized that my parents were going to eat the salad no matter what I said. There didn't seem to be anything I could do to warn or persuade them that I was almost, sort of, kind of positive that something was wrong with the food.

A short while later at dinner, I watched in terror as my parents ate the salad. My mom complimented me on the good job I had done preparing it. But the more I watched them eat, the sicker I felt. At first, I kept searching for a reason to explain why I had done such an awful thing. Eventually, though, I became resigned to the idea that I had just poisoned my parents. Otherwise, I reasoned, I wouldn't be so worried about it. At this point, I started to genuinely hate myself.

As I later discovered, this is a very common logical leap in OCD. People tell themselves that, if the thought weren't already true or about to be true, they wouldn't be anxious about it. They believe the anxiety is an indicator of probability—but it isn't. The anxiety is an alarm, but it's a false one.

Desperate and Despairing

The illness was chipping away at my ability to accomplish anything constructive in my daily life. I was taking medication and going to therapy, but treatment appeared to be doing far too little for me. Within the first year after my diagnosis, I had lost faith that things would work out for the better. I began to search for extreme ways out, and thoughts of suicide even crossed my mind.

I discussed how I was feeling with my psychiatrist. I felt safe in his office, and only his office, because I believed he had some sort of control over my actions. Surely, I thought, a psychiatrist was morally and legally bound to prevent me from doing anything that might bring harm to myself or my parents, as I had been afraid would happen. I communicated as much to him. He asked if I felt safe living at home, and although it was difficult to admit, I said that I really didn't.

Then came the night of the "poisoned" salad. Horrified by what I thought I had done, I finally ran from the dinner table screaming and broke down crying in the foyer. I could still smell dinner in the air, but my mind was on much less comforting subjects. For the life of me, I couldn't seem to get up off the floor, and soon I was sobbing harder than I had ever sobbed before.

My dad called the psychiatrist right then and there. Meanwhile, my mom held me close to her, trying to help me calm down and get a grip on my hysteria. Tears splashed down my cheeks and fell in streams onto the carpet. There was no way around it: I finally had to admit that I was out of control.

There was no way around it: I finally had to admit that I was out of control.

It took some time for me to feel confident that I could even walk from the house to the station wagon. I was petrified, and I couldn't think straight. Once in the car, we peeled off down the road and drove directly to my psychiatrist's office. He assessed me on the spot. I was at my lowest point. I was miserable, and I just wanted to feel safe. My psychiatrist nodded to me, and we both knew that a very important and rather devastating decision had just been made.

The room fluttered and blurred around me, and I began to sob quietly to myself. This was surrender, the moment when I realized that my life had become unmanageable and I needed the help of professionals who could watch me day and night. I curled up into a ball on the chair, with my knees tucked between my arms and my head rolling on the leather chair back. I concentrated on that leather smell, like a freshly cleaned car, and drifted off into my own thoughts.

When I returned to reality, my psychiatrist was talking on the phone. He identified himself and offered up a quick summary of my situation. Then he inquired about the number of available beds and asked if they could have one ready for me that night. After ending the call, he turned and informed me that there was a bed waiting for me at the psychiatric hospital.

Inside a Psych Ward

It wasn't until the adrenaline wore off that I actually understood what was going on. It's not that I was in a state of agitation or shock. I was just exhausted. I was tired of obsessing, tired of being afraid all the time—really, just tired in general. But when I found myself holding a pen in the hospital admissions office, I felt the full force of what I had agreed to.

My dad, ever cautious, pored over the stack of paperwork. He grimaced, and I could see that he had found something that he wasn't comfortable with. While he and the admissions lady talked about it, I stared off into space for a few moments, wondering what I was doing there. Then I began looking around the room for something to count. My stomach clenched into a tight ball, and I had an overwhelming desire for some fresh air and a soft bed to lie down in.

After the paperwork was completed and I had signed on the dotted line, I found out what a psychiatric hospital was really like. As I entered, the doors were locked behind me by key and access card. I was sealed inside. Then they asked me to check all my personal belongings. I didn't have much with me, but what few belongings I had all went into a small bag with my name on it. Once I had proved myself responsible enough, I might be allowed to look inside the bag and even take something out. But for now, the bag was stored at the nurse's station.

Next they took my bootlaces. Oddly enough, this was the first thing that really upset me. Looking back, I find this ironic, since I had so much trouble getting in and out of my boots anyway due to my obsessions and compulsions. Yet I was cognizant of the fact that there was something very serious about having my bootlaces confiscated. It meant the hospital staff didn't trust me. I realized this was because I had signed a waiver admitting that I didn't trust myself.

After that, I was issued a small bar of soap, washcloth, and towel. In addition, I was offered the choice of a razor. I found this funny for two reasons. First, I didn't have enough facial hair to making shaving a very productive activity. Second, it seemed ridiculous that they would take my bootlaces and give me a razor blade.

The shower that followed was very strange. A male orderly had to be inside the small bathroom with me, supervising as I washed myself. Not surprisingly, I felt embarrassed at first. But then I reasoned that I was doing something perfectly normal, just taking an ordinary shower. He was the one in the uncomfortable position of having to supervise. Looking at the situation that way helped a lot, and I even managed to make idle conversation with the orderly.

Once settled into the hospital, my days there were marked by regimen and routine. Medications were dispensed morning, noon, and night in small, wax-coated cups. Each time, I was given several pills to wash down with lukewarm water. Afterward I had to stick out my tongue to show that I had actually swallowed the pills. Then it was time to shuffle off to either my room or the common areas. All of the common areas, I noticed immediately, were alarmingly contaminated.

At the time of my hospitalization, there were very few inpatient programs geared specifically to OCD. As a result, I was lumped together with all the other psychiatric patients and treated the same way. I'll talk more about the benefits of OCD-specific programs in "The Big Picture" section below. Suffice it to say that my hospital stay wasn't optimal by current standards. In addition to drug therapy, the best programs today offer a form of psychotherapy that is specially designed to help people with OCD overcome obsessions and compulsions. I know this sounds odd, but sometimes I get a bit jealous of the superior options that people have now.

... the best programs today offer a form of psychotherapy that is specially designed to help people with OCD overcome obsessions and compulsions.

I can't promise that the food will be any better today, though. One thing that all psychiatric hospitals seem to have in common is gelatin desserts. Even if you don't like them now, should you ever go to the hospital, there's a good chance you'll have a taste for jiggly desserts by the time you're discharged.

The Big Picture

I have to press myself to recall the months just after my diagnosis, which culminated in a hospital stay. They were tumultuous times. I've since put twelve years between myself and those experiences, but the memories still hurt. Yet I know I must dig deep and make peace with my past. I do this for me, but I also do it for all of you who are feeling angry, sad, and scared. If sharing my experiences helps you cope with your own, then some good has come from my pain. This will heal me. This will make me stronger. And I hope that my strength, in turn, will support you.

In time, I moved past my anger and depression and found acceptance. There's a surprising measure of comfort in coming to terms with having OCD. By acceptance, I don't mean complacence, however. Under no circumstances would I urge you to simply "suck it up" and resign yourself to living with your obsessions and compulsions. To the contrary, I'm here to encourage you to take charge of your future. But to do that, you first need to identify and accept what's wrong.

What Are the Warning Signs?

Do you suspect that you might have OCD? No two individuals experience the disorder exactly the same way. However, these are some common warning signs:

- Having upsetting thoughts that keep coming back, even though you try to suppress them
- Being unusually worried about dirtiness or sinfulness

- Washing your hands, showering, or cleaning excessively
- Fearing contamination from shaking hands or touching everyday objects
- Doing things over and over a set number of times
- Growing increasingly preoccupied with minor details
- Checking repeatedly that the doors are locked or the stove is turned off
- Touching objects in a particular, repeated sequence
- Being very inflexible about how things are arranged
- Becoming distressed when objects aren't lined up properly or facing the right way
- Hoarding or collecting an excessive amount of junk
- Feeling as if daily life has become a great struggle

At some point, teens and adults with OCD realize that their intrusive thoughts and repetitive behaviors are getting out of hand. Yet they're unable to stop or ignore the thoughts and behaviors for long. Soon the obsessions and compulsions begin causing serious problems, often in several areas of life. As a result, OCD invariably leads to one or more of the following reactions:

- Emotional distress
- Time-consuming obsessions or compulsions that take up more than an hour a day
- Interference with usual activities or relationships
- Impaired ability to get along at school or work

THOUGHTS OF SUICIDE
It's very difficult to live, day in and day out, with disturbing thoughts or images. The difficulty is compounded when you don't understand what's causing the problem. If you don't

realize that your distressing thoughts are the result of a treatable illness, you may feel as if you'll never be able to escape them.

In the face of such pressure, some people have suicidal thoughts or impulses. Surprisingly little research has been done on the relationship between OCD and suicide. However, a large, national, three-year study of adults in the Netherlands found that having an anxiety disorder, such as OCD, increased the risk of later suicidal thoughts or suicide attempts. The increase wasn't due just to other mental disorders that sometimes occur along with anxiety, either. For example, people who had both an anxiety disorder and a mood disorder, such as depression, were more likely to attempt suicide than those who had a mood disorder alone.

While persistent suicidal thoughts and feelings aren't uncommon, they *are* a serious warning sign that should always be taken seriously. If you're thinking about suicide or feeling an urge to harm yourself, *get help immediately.* Tell a parent or another trusted adult how you're feeling. Talk to your doctor, therapist, or school counselor. Or call a suicide prevention hotline (see the box on the opposite page) and ask for a referral to resources in your community.

If not properly treated, OCD can make life lonely and miserable. At times, you may wonder whether it's even worth living. About this, I can assure you of two things. First, it's okay to feel this way. It shows that you have feelings that are as fragile and genuine as anyone else's. Second, no matter how much pain you may be feeling now, life can and will get better. At my lowest point, I was certain that my situation was hopeless. I was wrong. Remember

At my lowest point, I was certain that my situation was hopeless. I was wrong.

that I'm telling you this from the perspective of someone who has come through the darkness. At first, you may need to take it on faith, but there are brighter days waiting in your future, too.

Where Can I Turn for Help?

Just because you keep some quirky routines or act like a "neat freak" doesn't necessarily mean you have OCD. But if you recognize several of these warning signs in yourself, and if these thoughts and behaviors are making your life much less pleasant and rewarding, it may be time to seek help.

Your parents often are your biggest allies in finding a mental health professional who can diagnose and treat your problem. Just remember that, although some compulsive rituals are obvious to others, the obsessive thoughts underlying them are not. In order to help, your parents need to know what you've been going through, so start a frank discussion about what's troubling you.

If you're very, very lucky, your parents will get it right away and know exactly what to do. If that's not how it happens for you, though, try not to take it personally. It can be hard for parents to accept that their child has an illness. Plus, they may not know much about OCD in particular or mental illness in general. Sharing this book with your parents is one way to get

---

Call for Help

These national, 24-hour hotlines can provide immediate assistance if you ever find yourself thinking seriously about suicide:
- National Hopeline Network, 1–800–SUICIDE (784–2433)
- National Suicide Prevention Lifeline, 1–800–273-TALK (8255)

the ball rolling. You also can point them toward the other resources listed at the end of this book.

Besides your parents, you can ask your family doctor or
school counselor to help you find mental health care. Other
possible sources of referrals include a trusted teacher or your
school nurse or religious advisor. You also might try calling
your local mental health center, hospital, or medical school. If
one of your parents has an employee assistance program (EAP)
through work, that's another good starting point. In addition,
the federal government offers an online mental health services
locator at www.mentalhealth.samhsa.gov/databases.

MENTAL HEALTH PROFESSIONALS

Professionals from several different fields can diagnose and
treat OCD. The various fields have their own training and
licensure requirements, which may vary somewhat from state
to state. Following is a brief rundown of the different types of
medical and mental health professionals you might run into:

- *Psychiatrists* (M.D., D.O.) are medical doctors who
  specialize in the diagnosis and treatment of mental
  illnesses and emotional problems. While some psychiatrists provide therapy, many focus mainly on prescribing and monitoring medication, often working
  closely with therapists from other fields.
- *Other physicians* (M.D., D.O.) also can prescribe
  medication for OCD. However, they don't have specialized training in mental health care.
- *Psychologists* (Ph.D., Psy.D., Ed.D.) are mental health
  professionals who provide assessment and treatment
  for mental and emotional disorders. Treatment usually
  consists of therapy or other psychological techniques.

A few states allow psychologists with special training to write prescriptions.

- *Clinical social workers* (M.S.W., D.S.W., Ph.D.) are mental health professionals who are trained not only in therapy, but also in patient advocacy. Some provide assistance in getting help from government agencies.
- *Psychiatric nurses* (A.P.R.N.) are advanced practice registered nurses with specialized training in mental health care. In addition to providing therapy, psychiatric nurses can prescribe medication in many states.
- *Mental health counselors* (M.A., M.S., M.Ed., Ph.D., Ed.D.) are professionals who provide therapy and other mental health services. They typically combine traditional therapy with practical problem-solving techniques.

How Is a Diagnosis of OCD Made?

The first step toward freeing yourself from OCD is to get an accurate diagnosis. A mental health professional will ask you questions about your obsessions, compulsions, and overall well-being. Often, the questions are presented in a structured interview, in which the questions that are asked and the order in which they're presented are predetermined. The goal is to explore the nature of your symptoms, how severe they are, and how long they've lasted. This information can then be compared to diagnostic criteria in the *Diagnostic and Statistical Manual of Mental Disorders,* Fourth Edition, Text Revision (*DSM-IV-TR,* for short), a manual

> The first step toward freeing yourself from OCD is to get an accurate diagnosis.

published by the American Psychiatric Association. Mental health professionals from many fields use this manual for diagnosing all kinds of mental disorders. In addition to the verbal interview, you might be asked to fill out a paper-and-pencil questionnaire.

To find out more about your behavior at home as well as your mental, physical, and emotional development growing up, the mental health professional may ask your parents for information. To learn about how your symptoms are affecting you at school, the professional also might ask for permission to talk with your teachers.

It sounds straightforward enough. In reality, though, the process is complicated by the fact that several other disorders can resemble OCD. For instance, generalized anxiety disorder is another anxiety disorder that leads to excessive worry about a variety of things. The difference is that the concerns deal with real-life circumstances. In contrast, the obsessions of OCD usually have little basis in reality. But it's a subtle distinction that can be very difficult to make. That's where the professional's training and experience come into play.

What Kinds of Treatment Really Work?

Psychotherapy, or "talk therapy," is the cornerstone of treatment for OCD. But the type of psychotherapy that many people are familiar with—the type that focuses on gaining insight into past experiences and current emotional conflicts—hasn't proved to be very helpful. On the other hand, there's a large and growing body of evidence showing that another form of psychotherapy, called cognitive-behavioral therapy (CBT), can be quite effective. In CBT, the focus is on learning how to identify and change self-defeating thought patterns and maladaptive behaviors.

One particular type of CBT, called exposure and response prevention (EX/RP), has proved to be especially helpful for treating OCD. The "exposure" part involves having people confront the situations that lead to obsessing. This usually is done hierarchically; in other words, by gradually moving from situations that cause milder distress to those that cause more severe distress. The person with OCD and the therapist work together to agree upon the exposure hierarchy and to ensure that the treatment doesn't amount to too much, too fast.

This confrontation can occur either in real-life scenarios or in the imagination. The "response prevention" part involves voluntarily refraining from using compulsions to reduce distress during and after these encounters. When people repeatedly face their fears without resorting to compulsions, their anxiety gradually fades over time.

Many people with OCD also benefit from taking medication. In fact, the combination of CBT and medication can be more effective than either treatment by itself. The medications used to treat OCD are classified as antidepressants—in other words, medications used to prevent or relieve depression. However, they're widely prescribed to treat anxiety disorders as well.

SSRIs are antidepressants that increase the brain's supply of serotonin. Large, well-controlled studies have shown that various SSRIs are effective for treating OCD in children, adolescents, and adults. An older type of antidepressant called clomipramine (Anafranil) has been shown to work as well. Like the SSRIs, it affects the concentration and activity of serotonin in the brain.

Different people respond differently to therapy and medication, so treatment needs to be individualized. For example, if CBT alone doesn't provide enough relief, the treatment

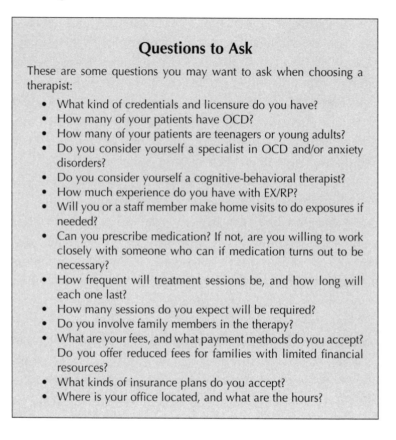

Questions to Ask

These are some questions you may want to ask when choosing a therapist:

- What kind of credentials and licensure do you have?
- How many of your patients have OCD?
- How many of your patients are teenagers or young adults?
- Do you consider yourself a specialist in OCD and/or anxiety disorders?
- Do you consider yourself a cognitive-behavioral therapist?
- How much experience do you have with EX/RP?
- Will you or a staff member make home visits to do exposures if needed?
- Can you prescribe medication? If not, are you willing to work closely with someone who can if medication turns out to be necessary?
- How frequent will treatment sessions be, and how long will each one last?
- How many sessions do you expect will be required?
- Do you involve family members in the therapy?
- What are your fees, and what payment methods do you accept? Do you offer reduced fees for families with limited financial resources?
- What kinds of insurance plans do you accept?
- Where is your office located, and what are the hours?

provider may change to more intensive CBT or add an SSRI. If the combination of intensive CBT and an SSRI isn't sufficient, the provider may switch to a different medication or add a second prescription. To learn more about the various treatment options, see Chapter 4.

When Is Hospitalization Helpful?

The vast majority of the time, treatment for OCD is provided on an outpatient basis. In other words, you stay at home, and you go to school or take part in your other activities as usual.

But you occasionally go to an office or clinic to see your doctor or therapist. The frequency of visits can range from several days a week to once a month or less, depending on how you're doing.

Occasionally, though, a short hospital stay may be the best and quickest way to get severe symptoms under control. Hospitalization involves inpatient treatment in a facility that provides intensive, specialized care and close, round-the-clock monitoring. It's the costliest and most restrictive form of mental health care, so it's reserved for the most severe or highest risk cases. If you have OCD, there's an excellent chance that hospitalization will never become an issue. But when you really need the extra care and attention, it can be invaluable.

> *Occasionally, a short hospital stay may be the best and quickest way to get severe symptoms under control.*

Decisions about hospitalization are made on a case-by-case basis. As examples, though, a hospital stay might be recommended if you:

- Are struggling with suicidal or aggressive impulses
- Are malnourished due to severe obsessions with food contamination
- Need close monitoring of your medication for a while
- Have not improved in treatment outside the hospital

One drawback is that there are only a few inpatient programs that are specifically designed for treating OCD in teenagers. Most general psychiatric units simply don't offer the EX/RP therapy that a teen with OCD needs. As a result, they may provide little help for coping with things that trigger obsessions once the teen leaves the hospital. In addition, traditional hospital programs often focus on strict adherence to rules and schedules, which may be nearly impossible for someone in the grips of severe OCD to follow. This failure to meet expectations may lead to more anxiety, not less. It also may heighten concerns about being "bad" or "crazy."

On the other hand, OCD-specific hospital programs provide intensive treatment including EX/RP and medication. When nothing else seems to work, they may offer the most improvement in the least amount of time, and the results are often long-lasting. If your doctor recommends hospitalization, ask whether the program is geared specifically toward treating OCD. Of course, even if there's no such program in your area, a short hospital stay still might be warranted to keep you safe and well. But when you have the option, choose an OCD-specific program.

What's the Least I Need to Know?

Relentless doubt is an integral part of OCD. In fact, dating back to the nineteenth century, the French have used the term *folie du doute* (doubting disease) for the disorder. Everyone worries from time to time about whether the door is locked or the food is safe to eat. But when you have OCD, the doubt never goes away for long. You're left with a nagging sense of unease and anxiety, and you wind up spending more and more time trying to assuage those feelings. Yet try as you might, the doubt always returns, because nothing is ever safe or clean enough.

It's not a fun way to live. But by recognizing that you have a problem, you've already started the process of finding a solution. A mental health professional can help you determine whether the culprit is actually OCD. If so, appropriate treat-

I Doubt It

Fifth grade was the year when I was forced to write exclusively with pens—the more indelible, the better. The homework assignments I turned in that year were torn up from cross-outs and corrections. That's when it first dawned on me how much of my time was spent on second-guessing and doubt. Nagging and incessant, impatient, and relentless doubt. It was like the dull throb after you cut your finger. The pain is always there in the background, but you're especially aware of it at certain, often inconvenient times.

As I write these paragraphs, I notice that I'm counting the words to make sure they equal a "good" number. This is the dull throbbing of OCD, the pang of constant uncertainty. It's there, but it's only ambient noise until a random word, sentence, or thought crosses from the subconscious to the conscious, making itself known. I've learned to recognize these recurring pangs of doubt for what they are; namely, pains in the ass, but pains that I've learned to live with and keep under control.

ment with therapy, medication, or both can help you break free from obsessive thoughts and time-consuming rituals. Although it's rarely needed, hospitalization is another option if the situation ever reaches a crisis point.

Of course, when you have a doubting disease, it's natural to doubt whether treatment really can make a difference. It can, although you may not notice a dramatic difference overnight. Our go-get-'em society often leads us to expect instant gratification. Unfortunately, treatment doesn't always work out that way. As a youngster newly diagnosed with OCD, I struggled with this reality. As a young adult who has regained control of his life, however, I can tell you that the time and effort you put into recovery will be repaid many times over.

Chapter Three

Adventures in Daily Living: OCD at Home and School

My Story

Locker rooms are full of disease, or at least they feel that way. So it's no surprise that one of the first times my OCD manifested itself at school involved a locker room. My classmates seemed to like it there. They ran around the room, squirting bottles of cologne at each other, telling tasteless jokes, and pelting each other with dirty clothes like a cotton snowball fight. But I hated that room. The smell of feet, sweat, and body odor was enough to make me gag.

Some days, the soccer team brought a sizable chunk of the field inside on their cleats, and the dank smell of earth added to the nauseating odors. I would look down and think about how many people had traveled that dirty floor. No matter how much the janitor cleaned, I was still anxious. To protect myself, I usually wore boots, which became my foot armor.

At the school I attended for three years beginning in middle school, gym was mandatory for everyone. Each student was assigned a locker with a combination lock. On the first day of gym class, your combination could be found on a piece of paper, like the fortune from a fortune cookie, taped to the lock.

Unfortunately, the combination was composed of three numbers that were arbitrary, not based on any number system in my head. And the knob on the lock had to be turned forward and backward in a pattern that was predetermined, not based on any pattern I felt compelled to follow. If I compulsively turned the knob too far, the tumblers in the lock wouldn't line up, and it wouldn't open. To make matters worse, even when compulsions weren't getting in my way, I had the hardest time figuring out which direction to turn the knob. I later learned that this was related to a math disability. I think everyone in my grade knew my locker combination within a month, because I had to ask for help with the lock so often.

I wasn't comfortable changing into my gym clothes. The idea of putting on a dirty t-shirt and gym shorts was gross. In addition, the thought of people watching me change clothes made me obsess over what they thought of me. And exposing body parts made me terrified that I would contract some airborne pathogen and fall violently ill. For all these reasons, I waited to change until the others had left the locker room to throw basketballs at each others' heads.

... the thought of people watching me change clothes made me obsess over what they thought of me.

I also had to dress according to very specific rules. If I put on my socks before my shorts, which I was prone to do because I was so repulsed by the dirty floor, then I would have to undress completely and start the process all over again. Needless to say, I was almost always late to gym class.

Locker Room Meltdown

One day, it went too far even by OCD standards—and that's far indeed. I was running later than usual, and everyone else had already scuttled out the double doors leading from the locker room. I began changing into my gym clothes, but somewhere along the line, the anxious thoughts looping through my brain took over, and I lost track of everything else. When I finally snapped out of it, I realized, much to my confusion and distress, that I wasn't wearing any clothes except my socks and shoes. Standing there nearly nude in the middle of the floor, I panicked.

I was terrified that the other students would return to change back into their regular clothes and find me still semi-naked. Yet I had to fight with my brain for several minutes to put on even a marginally decent number of clothes. Finally, I collapsed onto the floor, crying. Unable to shake my mind free from obsessions, I felt mentally stuck and physically rooted to the ground. Unless someone I trusted could assure me that it was perfectly fine to keep dressing, I wasn't going to budge from that spot. I needed reassurance from a person of authority that a cataclysm wasn't going to happen or, if it did, that it would have little or nothing to do with the way I got dressed.

Eventually, I started yelling to see if anyone—by that point, it didn't matter who—would hear me and come to bail me out from my personal jail. My voice became hoarse from yelling so much. I sobbed onto the dirty floor, and I wondered if I was doomed to stay on that nasty spot until I starved to death or caught some fatal illness from the filth.

At that moment, the coach happened to go into his office, and he heard me cry out. He came into the locker room, concerned and confused. Although he didn't know much about

OCD, the coach, like all the faculty, was aware that I had something wrong with my head, that I would get scared for no apparent reason, and that I would often need the help of adults, whether I liked it or not.

Looking back, I think the coach must have been considering the rules about contact with a student, as it was rather obvious that what I really needed was a hug. In the end, I think he weighed the risk and decided to hell with it. He came over, knelt beside me, and wiped my tears until I looked up in choking sobs. Then he asked me what had happened. To be honest, I didn't really know, and I told him as much.

Just Following Orders

I wonder in retrospect how that must have sounded. I was crying on a grimy locker room floor, disoriented and anxious. Unaware of how I had reached the point of immobility, I was still clinging to the orders in my head that said to stay put until someone else told me what to do.

I cried for a long time. Another student—a good-hearted friend who cared about my condition and wanted to help—wandered into the locker room. Ironically, I think he was hoping to skip out of extra laps around the gym for some insubordination. Luckily for him, good Samaritans are more in demand than discipline cases. The coach told my friend to contact the other gym teachers and explain that the boys' locker room was temporarily closed and gym students would be excused from other classes until they could change.

The coach sat with me and coached me through getting dressed. He assured me that no harm would befall me or any-one else if I opened my locker and finished putting on my clothes. When I was finally dressed, I felt a ripple of fatigue wash through my body. It's incredibly draining to put that much effort into anything. I collapsed against the coach and cried. He asked what else he could do to help, and I thanked God for this man who had wandered through by sheer providence and helped me overcome the immobilizing effects of anxiety.

At last, I was ready to leave. Unseen by the other students, I exited the locker room and went to my advisor's office, where I could catch my breath and get my bearings. After I was gone, the locker room was reopened. My classmates changed into their regular clothes without ever realizing how close they had come to witnessing one of my less-than-stellar moments. That was the scariest part of the whole disease for me. OCD was unpredictable, awkward, and embarrassing. It would crop up in the most inconvenient places—although I think it's safe to say there's really no such thing as a good place for an OCD attack.

Retracing My Steps

I was extremely conscious of how my junior high school was physically laid out, and more specifically, of every path I took to navigate the hallways. At the start of each day, I knew exactly what route I would take and just how far I would have to travel. This was because I had counted the steps. I knew the exact number of steps required to get from one point to another, sorted by floors, grades, and subjects. If I failed to walk the correct number of paces from one doorway to the next, the whole plan was ruined, and I had to start over. As a result, I spent far more time than I would have liked pacing the halls, trying to hit the perfect stride. After the first month or so, I stopped paying attention to the puzzled looks of other students.

Crossing through doorways had to be done perfectly. It was absolutely essential that the correct foot pass through first. This was more difficult than it might sound, and if the incorrect foot was poised to cross the threshold, I had to do a little shuffle to make the steps come out right.

Every afternoon, I would mentally review the entire day's foot traffic route and come up with a path to finish off the day correctly. The path would occasionally—although thankfully, not often—lead me outdoors, down to the swing sets or monkey bars, and through the track field until I reached one of the more obscure entrances to the school building.

Even while seated at my desk during class, I was preoccupied with such thoughts. Often I sat there mentally optimizing my escape route after class was over. By the time the bell actually rang, I was exhausted by the effort of sorting through innumerable alternatives to find the best one. Yet no matter how meticulously I followed the chosen path, I never felt satisfied, because the rules that governed my compulsive walking kept getting more and more demanding.

I never felt satisfied, because the rules that governed my compulsive walking kept getting more and more demanding.

Like most students, the less I liked a class, the more trouble I had paying attention. This left my mind free to invent high-anxiety obsessions and complicated compulsions. In particular, I tended to ruminate about disease and all the ridiculous responsibilities I had to protect other people. I realized that these "responsibilities" were the products of an OCD mind, not actual superpowers, but they still dominated my thoughts.

Math class was the worst. Leaving class, I might feel compelled to walk only along the cracks of the linoleum one day and only on the tiles the next. When I tried to figure out the reasons, I just became obsessed with obsessing. And so it went.

The more I resisted, the worse things got. The more I gave in, the worse things got. My mind was stuck in a lose-lose situation.

Paying Scrupulous Attention

I was raised primarily Jewish. When I was young, I enjoyed going to temple. The idea of a loving God smiling down on humanity made me feel secure and less alone. After my diagnosis with OCD, though, I wasn't so sure. Why, I wondered, had God let this happen to me? Surely I had done something wrong, but what? I had been a good kid, as far as I knew. I did my best to stay out of trouble. I was smart and engaging, and I tried to make others happy. To me, this whole ordeal seemed as if it had befallen the wrong person, and I was pretty mad about that.

One religious holiday in particular stands out in my memories from this time. Yom Kippur, the Jewish day of repentance, is considered one of the holiest days of the year. It's meant to be a time of atonement and reconciliation, but for me, it was simply agony.

Sitting in temple in a folding chair that had been pulled out of storage for the huge Yom Kippur turnout, I listened as the rabbi recounted the atrocities committed upon the Israelites by the Pharaohs, the Romans, and, worst of all, the Nazis. The goal was to underscore just how far man can deviate from what is right and what is just. To guard against such deviance in oneself, all actions must be preceded by careful forethought and benevolence toward humankind. As someone with OCD, however, many of my actions were already preceded by hours or even days of forethought and scrutiny. It was my job to save the world on a daily basis, and the extra reminder of Yom Kippur only added to the overwhelming pressure.

One passage in the readings never failed to grab my attention. It referred to the Book of Life, in which God records the names and lives of the righteous. Meanwhile, the names of the unrighteous are blotted out, and I was certain that would be my fate. No matter how good a person I tried to be, I was sure I had angered God and would be punished for it. The reading of that particular passage always made my stomach want to play show and tell with those sitting next to me.

These thoughts of fault—these beliefs that God was angry with me and that I would always be out of favor—stemmed from scrupulosity. In this form of OCD, obsessive thoughts about offending God or being sinful often lead to so much praying that it becomes debilitating. I was a prime example.

No one else in the synagogue prayed harder than I did. I can say this with confidence, because I would pray for the entire service while simultaneously listening to the sermon and occasionally taking quick walks outside to catch my breath whenever I felt too anxious or sick. Yet I worried that the very act of walking out of the service was reason enough to anger God.

Sorry for Everything

My prayers were apologies, all of them. I apologized not for things I had actually done, but rather for unclean thoughts and violent images that intruded upon my mind. I apologized for not being loyal to Judaism all the time, for having doubts, and for spurning God for what I felt he had done to me. The observances lasted several hours, but my prayers went on for much longer than that. I didn't understand why, no matter how much I prayed, the OCD didn't wane. The more I sought God's forgiveness, the more I found flaw with my prayers.

Dialogue on the Damned

When I was in college, I was lucky enough to see a psychiatrist who had been an ordained priest in a previous life. Eventually, I worked up the courage to ask a question I had on my lips, even though I was afraid and embarrassed to admit it: "What if I make God angry here?"

I was thinking about some of my therapy sessions, which involved exposing myself to music that I was sure would earn me poor favor with God. Yet I clearly had some issues with music to work out. I had bought a CD by a group called The Damned, for instance, but I had to quarantine the CD under lock and key in my dorm until God let me listen to it.

"God wants you to get better," Dr. Q. told me. "If your treatment requires you to say or do things that might otherwise seem like heresy, so be it. If you accept that God is the definitive divine power, then you must also accept that he understands things we mortals do not."

"What will he understand about me?" I asked, fear trickling down my spine.

Dr. Q. replied, "He'll see that you're doing the work you need to do to get better."

"And if I offend him?"

"You won't."

"But what if I do?"

"That's my point," Dr. Q. said. "Human beings aren't perfect, but God loves us all. When we do the things we have to do to make ourselves and our lives better, we're doing what God wants."

I'd love to tell you that this one dialogue was enough to cure my scrupulosity. It wasn't. But it did give me something to think about and helped sustain me as I tackled scrupulosity in therapy.

When the rabbi brought out the Torah, bound in sheepskin and clad in gold and jewels, I was afraid to look at it. I felt that this was an object too holy for me to be around. I was too unclean, too marked, and too hated by God to be in the presence of his teachings. Sweat trickled down my neck and soaked my armpits, and my hands began to shake. Everyone else was there because they were good Jewish people. I was there to ruin everything, and in my mind, that's what I did.

When I was no longer able to handle the service, I would pick up the prayer book and read through it feverishly, hoping to temporarily escape the limelight of holy scrutiny. But the God I read about in those pages sometimes seemed vengeful and angry. After all, he did turn Lot's wife into a pillar of salt and unleash a rain of fire over Sodom and Gomorrah. I found little solace there.

After the service, it was a tradition to turn to the person standing next to you, ask for forgiveness, and grant forgiveness to that individual in turn. The mutual exchange of apology and forgiveness ended with wishes for a good year as well as much hugging and crying for joy. It should have been a warm, fuzzy moment. But I felt that my pleas for forgiveness were too little, too late. When my mother hugged me and told me how much she loved me, I would cry softly for all the pain I had caused her in the past and would surely bring her in the future.

The Big Picture

As I'm writing this book, more than ten years after my diagnosis, I feel as if I'm finally starting to get the hang of living with OCD. It's like a bad roommate. I'll never be thrilled about sharing my life with this disorder, but I'm learning how to get along with it.

I feel as if I'm finally starting to get the hang of living with OCD.

OCD can touch virtually every facet of day-to-day life. At home, it can turn the simplest tasks—such as taking a shower, getting dressed, or eating a meal—into terrible ordeals. The inflexible and often inexplicable nature of compulsions also can put a severe strain on family relationships. When one member of a family spends hours locked in the bathroom washing, goes through elaborate rituals before each meal, or becomes very upset when personal possessions are moved even slightly, it affects the quality of life for the rest of the family as well.

At school, obsessions sometimes become so distracting that it's nearly impossible to think about anything else. Meanwhile, compulsions can interfere both directly and indirectly with school performance. In my case, rituals dictating how I dressed for gym and walked through the halls often made me late for class. Other students might feel as if they must read each word in an assignment a specific number of times or retrace their handwriting until it is perfect. It's easy to see how such behaviors could make it hard to finish assignments on time.

Some teenagers with mild to moderate OCD are able to suppress most of their symptoms while at school. They feel the anxiety building up, but they struggle mightily to resist it because they fear embarrassment in front of their friends. By the time they get home, though, the pent-up symptoms usually are ready to bust out. Such teens may seem like different people at home than they are at school, leading their parents to suspect that they're just being manipulative or rebellious. In truth, the difference in behavior is a sign that they see home as a safer and less threatening place than school—a place where they can finally let out their anxiety.

If this is your pattern, there's a good chance it's causing some tension at home. Put yourself in your parents' shoes. It's not hard to see why they might feel confused by your behavior. Some may even think OCD turns on and off like a faucet in response to what you do and don't want to do. Of course, you know otherwise. If it were that easy, you could shut off OCD before it made you miserable. Talking honestly with your parents is one way to see each other's point of view. It also may help for your therapist to join in the conversation as a neutral and knowledgeable third party.

How Does OCD Affect Life at Home?

Living with OCD is stressful, whether you have the disorder yourself or simply share your home with someone else who does. Your family members may feel frustrated by their inability to change your patterns of behavior, especially those that are wreaking havoc with daily life. Meanwhile, you may feel guilty about being the source of so much distress. Unfortunately, anxiety about hurting your loved ones can make the symptoms worse, and that only increases the distress for all concerned. It's a destructive cycle that can tear a family apart if allowed to continue unchecked.

Fortunately, the picture doesn't have to be so bleak if you keep the lines of communication open. While it can be difficult to share what you are thinking and feeling, there's no way your parents can understand what you are going through if you don't tell them. Once you get your fears, anxieties, and "crazy" thoughts out in the open, you may find that simply exposing them to the light of day makes them less scary.

The first few conversations are apt to be the hardest, especially if your parents aren't familiar with OCD. In addition to talking about your thoughts and feelings, it helps to share information and resources. Then be prepared to listen as well as talk. Chances are, your parents have many questions and concerns of their own, and having an opportunity to air their thoughts and feelings about your behavior will be a relief for them, too. Over time, the conversations will probably get easier as you and your parents become more comfortable with the idea of OCD.

What if communication isn't exactly your family's strong point? You're certainly not alone. Try to see things from your parents' viewpoint. They may come from a background where feelings were swept under the rug rather than talked about openly. Or they may be having trouble accepting that their child has a chronic disease. They might not know much about mental illness. Or they might have a different perspective from yours because they have more life experience.

Each family's situation is a little different. But one thing they have in common is that, underneath any emotional distance or turmoil, the majority of parents want what's best for their child. If you suspect that OCD might be at the root of some problems, ask your parents to help you find professional help. Besides addressing the OCD symptoms, a therapist may be able to help your family work on developing better communication skills, if that's an ongoing challenge.

... underneath any emotional distance or turmoil, the majority of parents want what's best for their child.

DISABLING THE ENABLERS

Sometimes family members help perpetuate the ill person's OCD symptoms without meaning to do so. Therapy can help families identify and break free from such negative behavior patterns. In my case, as relationships at home grew more strained in my teens, my parents decided that we should try family therapy, in which the whole family takes part in therapy sessions together.

Every Saturday for a year was forfeit to these sessions. They always began with me talking about events in the previous week. I would implore the therapist to listen to me, and he did.

Unfortunately, he also listened to my parents and even my sister, which meant I often was forced to hear how my behavior affected those around me.

One purpose of these visits was to help my parents draw the line when it came to my compulsive rituals. Like many sympathetic family members, my parents sometimes went along with the rituals because they wanted to relieve my anxiety and keep the peace. Yet by cooperating with OCD, they were unintentionally doing their part to keep the rituals going. In therapy, my parents came to see that the best way to help was *not* to help with compulsive rituals, no matter how upset I got. After that, whenever I engaged in OCD behavior, I was on my own.

In hindsight, I understand why this was necessary. At the time, however, I found it a very bitter pill to swallow. The way I saw it, my parents should do everything in their power to help me feel better. If that meant checking a dozen times to make sure the lights were turned off, so be it. It wasn't until later that I was able to understand that the more my parents went along with my demands, the more of a hold OCD had not only on me, but also on my whole family.

How Does OCD Affect Life at School?

While some students with OCD manage to hide their symptoms at school, others have real difficulty meeting academic demands or getting along with their classmates. Common problems at school include:

- Lack of concentration. It's hard to listen in class, follow directions, or focus on assignments with a mind that is already filled with intrusive, obsessive thoughts.
- Social isolation. Compulsive rituals can lead to decidedly odd-looking behavior, and classmates are not always kind

or understanding. In addition, some teens with OCD pull back from their classmates rather than risk rejection or embarrassment.

- Low self-esteem. This is a common problem among teens with OCD, many of whom feel great shame, guilt, or distress over their symptoms. Their lack of self-confidence can undermine how well they do in academics, sports, and social activities.
- Medication side effects. The medications used to treat OCD occasionally cause side effects such as sleepiness, restlessness, or irritability. These side effects, in turn, may lead to disruptive behavior in class or interfere with a student's ability to learn.

Just as at home, communication is the key to managing OCD at school. If you think your symptoms are affecting your school performance, talk to your teachers or the school counselor about what's going on. Often relatively small changes can make a big difference in your ability to succeed at school.

In my case, I was allowed to go from class to class at my own pace. Although some of the other students saw this as an unfair privilege, I told myself that they didn't know what having OCD was like. Under the circumstances, a little extra time to walk through the hallways seemed like a reasonable compromise with the disorder.

Be prepared to educate the educators, since many may have little, if any, experience with OCD. To introduce the disorder, it may help for your parents to request a meeting with your teachers and other school staff. A parent-teacher meeting to discuss your behavior might sound like the kiss of death, but this is one instance when it could work to your advantage. Ask if you can be at the meeting, too. In addition, because OCD is a complicated subject, some families invite their therapist to attend the meeting or write a report to be read there.

At times, you, your parents, your teachers, and school administrators may not see eye-to-eye. That's understandable, since you each have slightly different perspectives. Ultimately, though, you all want the same thing: for you to be as successful as possible at school. The more you can work together as a team, the better the chances that this goal will be realized. A cooperative attitude on your part can go a long way toward enlisting the rest of the team's support.

What Steps Help Manage OCD at School?

There's no such thing as a one-size-fits-all solution to OCD problems at school. The classroom modifications that work well for one student might not be very helpful for you. The first thing you and your team need to do is identify the most appropriate strategies for addressing your particular needs.

There's no such thing as a one-size-fits-all solution to OCD problems at school.

Involving your therapist helps ensure that everyone is on the same page—and that helps maximize the benefits of both therapy and any changes you make at school.

Some teens find that it helps to have a designated "safe" place, such as the counselor's office, where they can go when their anxiety becomes overwhelming. Others find that being allowed to leave the classroom to get a drink or run an errand helps clear their thoughts when obsessions threaten to take over. You and your teachers might want to work out a private signal you can use when you need to be excused for this type of short break. Using the signal not only saves you embarrassment, but also minimizes the disruption for the rest of the class.

Other modifications are geared to coping with specific symptoms. Following are examples of the kinds of classroom changes that some students with OCD have found helpful. As treatment progresses, the need for many of these changes may gradually lessen and eventually disappear.

If you have handwriting compulsions (for example, writing and rewriting, erasing compulsively, or retracing the shape of letters)

- Printing, if cursive handwriting is the problem
- Taping lectures instead of taking notes
- Taking tests orally or on a computer
- Substituting projects for written assignments

If you have reading compulsions (for example, reading and rereading, or counting letters, words, or lines as you're reading)

- Listening to assigned books on tape
- Having someone else read to you
- Photocopying the reading assignment, and drawing a thick, black line through passages as you read them to prevent rereading

If you're bothered by contamination obsessions and washing compulsions

- Getting permission to be first in line at the cafeteria
- Sitting where you'll be the first to receive handouts
- Working out a policy with your teachers on bathroom access. (For some students, being allowed to go to the bathroom whenever they wish actually reduces the amount of time spent obsessing over cleanliness. For other students, especially as treatment progresses, limit-

ing bathroom access may be the best policy. Talk to your therapist and teachers about the best strategy for you.)

If you're slowed down by obsessions, compulsions, and perfectionism

- Making check marks instead of filling in circles on tests, if you have a compulsive need to fill in the circles perfectly
- Being allowed extra time for tests
- Setting time limits for homework. (For instance, a teacher might require you to spend a certain amount of time—and no more—on a homework assignment rather than having to answer a set number of questions.)

As you get better with treatment, you may be able to phase out many of these steps. Your therapist can help you determine when you're ready to start the phase-out process. In addition, your therapist can provide suggestions for easing out gradually so that you don't lose the progress you've made.

What Should You Tell Friends About OCD?

OCD may lead you to act in ways that your friends find puzzling, to say the least. If they don't know what's causing the behavior, they may conclude that you're spoiled, hard to get along with, or just plain weird. It's always your decision whether or not to tell friends about your disorder, though. If you do decide to talk with them, it's up to you how much information to share and when to broach the topic.

On one hand, not everyone needs to know the details of your personal life. In addition, some people are less than

Your Educational Rights

Some students with OCD need little, if any, help to get along well at school. Others, however, need more extensive changes in the classroom or special educational services. If your symptoms are causing serious problems at school, there are two federal laws applying to high school and younger students that you should know about: the Individuals with Disabilities Education Improvement Act of 2004 (IDEA) and Section 504 of the Rehabilitation Act of 1973. (For information about your educational rights as a college student, see the Frequently Asked Questions section at the end of this book.)

- IDEA—To qualify for services under IDEA, you must show that you have a disability that impacts your ability to benefit from general educational services. This requires going through an evaluation and being labeled with a disability such as "emotional disturbance" or "other health impairment." The process is lengthy and involved, so it's only appropriate if you have extensive, long-lasting needs. If you qualify, you'll receive an individualized education program (IEP)—a written educational plan that spells out how your individual needs will be met. For more details, visit the Web sites of the U.S. Department of Education (www.idea.ed.gov) or the Parent Advocacy Coalition for Educational Rights (www.pacer.org).
- Section 504—To qualify for services under Section 504, you must have a physical or mental impairment that substantially limits one or more major life activities. The 504 process is faster and more flexible than the one required under IDEA, and in many cases, it has less stigma attached to it. However, IDEA is usually a better choice for students with extensive special needs.

enlightened when it comes to mental illness. There might be some backlash, such as gossip or teasing. On the other hand, the only way to overcome the stigma attached to mental illness is by educating people, and one of the best ways of doing that is simply by sharing your story. While you might run into some mean-spirited responses, you're also likely to encounter many compassionate ones. True friends will understand your situation and be there for you, but they can't read your mind. To support you, they need to know what's going on.

Decide in advance how you'll handle the subject. For instance, when talking to close friends and classmates, you'll probably want to refer to OCD by name and take time to describe what the disorder is all about. You might add something like, "I'm receiving treatment, and it's helping, but getting better is a long-term process. I'd really appreciate your support." When questioned by strangers or casual acquaintances, though, you might not want to get into such a lengthy

---

Poster Child for OCD

On one occasion when I was about 15, I walked into Starbucks for a caffeine fix, cigarette dangling from my mouth. The mother of one of my childhood friends was there, and she stared at me strangely. I was suddenly very self-conscious. I thought maybe I was going to get another anti-smoking lecture (which, for the record, I should have listened to). But then she smiled, and my heartbeat slowed down a little as I realized that I wasn't in trouble after all.

My friend's mother said she was astonished to see that I was okay and "out and about," as she put it. I blinked back at her, wondering what the heck she was talking about. As we continued chatting, it turned out that she had heard I was very sick and assumed the worst. I was glad that my presence in Starbucks that day helped set the record straight, at least for her.

I still run into this reaction occasionally. Now that I'm in my twenties, I'll bump into someone I know as I'm on my way to work, wearing a suit and an ID badge, and I'll get the same astonished response. I've had more than one person tell me they're surprised to see that I've made it as far as I have. I choose to take such remarks as compliments, because I know that's how they're intended. I like to think that some people look at me and change their preconceived ideas about what young people with mental illness can—and cannot—accomplish. I didn't ask to be my community's poster child for OCD, but it's a role I've learned to accept and appreciate.

discussion. One option might be simply to say that you have OCD—or a "brain disorder" or "neurological condition"—and leave it at that.

The good news is that people generally are more familiar with OCD today than they were when I was first diagnosed years ago. At the time, attention-deficit hyperactivity disorder (ADHD)—a disorder characterized by a short attention span, overactivity, and/or impulsive behavior—was getting a lot of media attention, and many people confused OCD with ADHD. Others thought OCD was a form of schizophrenia, a severe mental illness that causes symptoms such as hearing voices that aren't there, distortions of perception, and irrational behavior. And still others regarded *any* mental illness as a shameful secret or taboo subject.

Slowly but surely, these kinds of misconceptions are being dispelled. You can do your part by sharing information when it feels appropriate. The more people know, the more they'll come to see that having OCD is similar to having asthma or diabetes. It's a challenging illness, but also a treatable one. And there's no reason it has to keep you from leading a "normal" life—whatever that means.

The more people know, the more they'll come to see that having OCD is similar to having asthma or diabetes.

What's the Least I Need to Know?

OCD is a multifaceted disorder that can affect multiple aspects of your life. Left unchecked, it can do serious harm to your personal relationships, home life, and school performance. Yet you have the power to write a happier ending to your story. The symptoms of OCD can be managed with proper treatment and self-care. Until your symptoms are completely under control, you still may have to contend with some OCD-related problems at home and school. But you can minimize these problems and prevent other ones by taking appropriate action.

Communication is critical. You're probably confused or disturbed by some of the behaviors you feel driven to repeat, even though you're privy to all the thoughts and feelings underlying these rituals. Imagine how much more confusing your behavior seems to someone who isn't inside your head. By sharing your thoughts and feelings with those who have your best interests at heart, you go a long way toward getting the help and support you need to overcome OCD.

Chapter Four

Reaching for a Lifeline: Psychotherapy and Medication

My Story

There came a point where psychotherapy just wasn't enough. That isn't to say that there weren't benefits, but my relationship with my therapist had evolved into a sort of outpouring of all my frustrations and rage. I would often come into his office, already steaming mad and with a laundry list of things that I was upset about. The idea of adjusting to a life where I had to deal with things that others my age didn't was enough to make me angry, confused, and rebellious. I cried a lot, I punched the pillows in his office, and I spent a lot of time engaging in behaviors that were, at their best, destructive.

One day, during a family vacation, I was watching the television while my sister longed to go to the beach. What I didn't know was that upstairs my mother and father were discussing how to break the news to me that I was going to a boarding school starting that fall.

My dad came down the stairs and informed me that we were having a family meeting, which, I have to tell you, wasn't exactly something that our family did very often. I wandered up the stairs with trepidation, wondering what I was about to find out. It turns out that for a little while now my family had been conspiring with my psychotherapist to find a boarding school that would provide a therapeutic atmosphere. What was worst of all was that I didn't even have a choice in the matter. The idea that I was going to live around a bunch of people in the same depressing situation as I, caged up until I could sort myself out, was horrifying. It was also at this time that I realized I was truly living a life that was unmanageable.

I didn't talk very much to my family for the remainder of that vacation. I simply sat in the living room and pouted. I was miserable. Everything I had known seemed far away, like it was slipping from my grasp, and I didn't think I was going to be able to conquer the next challenge.

Off to Boarding School

The first time I visited the boarding school that had been hand-picked for me, it was clear that the staff was already sizing me up to decide where to put me—and I'd thought I was just interviewing with the admissions counselor. A few weeks later, I was on my way to the school as an enrolled student. It was pouring rain that day. For the entire car ride there, I intentionally jacked up the volume on my music so high that it interfered with my parents' attempts at conversation. I wondered about the odds of survival if I made a daring escape via tuck and roll out the car door onto the highway. Such thoughts occupied my mind until we pulled up to the dorm that was to be my home for the next two years.

The first thing the school staff did was to explain the daily routine. Within a week or so, I started to get the hang of things. I got up in the morning and made my bed (which was harder than it sounds as I had the top bunk). I did my chore for the day—cleaning the bathrooms or sweeping the floors or vacuuming the halls. Then I tooled off to breakfast, followed by school.

At some point during the day, I would be paged to the office of Dr. Z, the psychologist, for a session. At first, I just vented my anger and frustration, but eventually I confided that OCD was really beating up on me and I needed help. Having seized up for so long, not open to any of the therapeutic possibilities presented to me, this was something new. I asked Dr. Z. what I should do next.

Somewhat to my surprise, he didn't gloat or say that I had just been stubborn all along. Instead, he asked me what was going on—what was happening inside my head, what I was afraid of, and what I was doing about it as far as my behavior went. His interest and concern were mind-blowing, to the point where it felt as if my brain actually blew across the room and slammed smack into the opposite wall. Here was a man who really understood what I was up against.

I eventually started to speak freely about whatever was on my mind. The thoughts often poured out as disconnected bits and pieces, and Dr. Z. would help me reassemble them into cohesive thought patterns. He often did this while we drove around in his convertible, which was really cool. As we weren't allowed to leave campus except under specific circumstances, this made therapy seem like a sort of vacation. I learned to look forward to getting the help I needed.

Hitting the Panic Button

Around this time, though, another issue became more and more pressing by the day: I was starting to have frequent panic attacks. A panic attack is a sudden, unexpected wave of intense fear and apprehension that's accompanied by physical symptoms, such as a rapid heart rate, shortness of breath, or sweating. In my case, my breath felt like it was being forcibly pushed out of me, and my heart pounded like I was running on a treadmill turned up to high speed while drinking coffee. My vision also would blur, and I would become disoriented.

These panic attacks often occurred at times when I couldn't get a handle on my OCD thoughts, allowing them to spiral out of control. The psychiatrist on campus suggested that I go on an anti-anxiety medication called Ativan (lorazepam). Because it's fast-acting, I could use Ativan on an as-needed basis, which meant that I only took it when I was having a severe

OCD + Another Anxiety Disorder

It's estimated that 40% of people with OCD will have another anxiety disorder at some point in their lives. The most common of these coexisting anxiety disorders are:

- Panic disorder—Characterized by the repeated occurrence and persistent fear of spontaneous panic attacks. The fear stems from the belief that such attacks will result in a catastrophe, such as having a heart attack.
- Generalized anxiety disorder—Characterized by excessive worry over a variety of things that are related to real-life circumstances.
- Social anxiety disorder—Characterized by marked fear in social situations that involve being around unfamiliar people or the possibility of scrutiny by others.

panic attack. But while Ativan provided a quick rescue from intense panic, the underlying OCD thoughts would still bubble up to the surface.

It was around this point that I learned about a plan for me to start seeing yet another therapist soon. This therapist specialized in cognitive-behavioral therapy (CBT), which focuses on identifying and changing maladaptive thought and behavior patterns. I have to say, I wasn't too interested in CBT when I first heard about it. I was still hoping for a pill—or a cocktail of pills—that would fix me up and make everything better.

Besides, I was afraid to tackle CBT. The most effective form of CBT for treating OCD is something called exposure and response prevention, which involves confronting the situations that lead to obsessing while refraining from using compulsions to reduce distress during these encounters. That sounded like heavy-duty treatment to me, and I wasn't sure I was ready for it. The way it was described to me didn't help. I heard words like "painful," "sweating," and "anxious"—probably not the best way to introduce a therapeutic option. It took two years before I finally agreed to give CBT a try.

Winning by Surrender

In the meantime, my whole life seemed to spin out of control. My self-esteem plummeted, my will to live dropped to a new low, and I was smoking instead of eating. My weight fluctuated with the frequency of the New England weather. Throughout this whole time, I knew that the way to make a positive change in my life was by consenting to CBT. Yet I refused to do it.

These days, parents of young people diagnosed with OCD often ask me what they can do to get their kids to participate fully in therapy. I tell these parents that they have to accept their powerlessness over the situation. As devastating and bleak as this advice may sound at first, it's crucial to being a supportive parent. From your point of view, the message is equally stark: No one—not even your parents—can force recovery onto you. They can only encourage and foster it. It's up to you to approach therapy with an open mind and a willingness to work hard at getting better.

Left to its own devices, OCD will run rampant through a person's life, doing all kinds of damage. My life became unmanageable. Compulsive rituals transformed something as simple as taking a shower into sheer torture. Meanwhile, harming obsessions made me so afraid of hurting someone that I spent as much time as possible by myself indoors. I gave up on trying.

Eventually, though, the day came when I was so exhausted and frustrated that I could no longer deny the obvious: What I was doing wasn't working. Angry and a bit sad, I stubbed out my cigarette in the dirt and put my head in my hands. I decided at that moment that I needed more than a quick fix. To use the terminology of recovery, I surrendered to my situation. I didn't want to be sick anymore, but the disease was all I knew, and I realized that I was unable to fight it alone. It was a staggering realization, and I cried until my eyes were almost too slippery to stay inside their sockets.

That day, I gave in. I requested a meeting with the psychologist and let him know that I was ready to try CBT. If you ever find yourself in this situation, don't expect it to be easy. Admitting first to yourself and

Admitting first to yourself and then to someone else that you cannot beat OCD single-handedly is one of the hardest things in the world.

then to someone else that you cannot beat OCD single-handedly is one of the hardest things in the world. But if you're struggling, it's also the best thing you can possibly do for yourself.

The psychologist called my parents, who were elated by my change of heart. Soon I was riding in my dad's car to meet the new cognitive-behavioral therapist. That car trip followed the same pattern as others to come: I got into the passenger seat, took a sedative, put the seat down, and listened to music. I remember staring at the trees as we drove past, noting how the foliage fluttered and flickered.

When we arrived at the cognitive-behavioral therapist's home, which doubled as his office, we found ourselves parking in a meadow. Rustic farm tools rested on an old wall that was hand-crafted out of stone and mortar. Yet despite the peaceful surroundings, a sense of unease came over me as I stumbled out of the car.

The therapist stuck out his hand, and when I shook it, he leaned in to meet me the way a person greets someone he already knows and cares about. Then he led me toward the nicely furnished office in the basement. When he gestured toward a chair across from his, I sat down and waited to see what would happen.

Dr. C. asked about my symptoms, and I told him, only partly joking, that I had all of them. That seemed to effectively encapsulate my situation, I thought. Then I told him about the checking, counting, cleanliness obsessions, harming obsessions, intrusive thoughts, disabling fears—anything that seemed at all useful. Dr. C. busily took notes the whole time I was talking. While I had no way of knowing it at the time, I had just taken a giant step down the path toward recovery.

Cognitive-Behavioral Help

Because I was still living at the therapeutic boarding school, I was lucky enough to have several treatment providers working together on my behalf during this time. At home, I still had my original psychiatrist, who oversaw my treatment and reviewed any medication changes. At school, I had another psychiatrist as well as a psychologist with whom I could explore what was going on in my life. And now I had a new cognitive-behavioral therapist with whom I could really hammer away at the OCD symptoms. Although having so many treatment providers may sound over the top, I think the team approach helped a lot.

My CBT sessions were intense. The sessions, which were actually a series of lessons, had me tackling my symptoms hands-on. The first word in CBT is cognitive, and the first thing I learned in therapy was how to sort out my thinking. Obsessions are sly by nature. They infiltrate trains of thought and disguise themselves to appear just like the other thoughts. CBT teaches you to ferret out the obsessive thoughts and rip away their camouflage. Once you unmask a thought as obsessive—in other words, as nothing more than the absurd masquerading as the usual and the rational—you take away much of its power to cause distress.

The next thing I learned was how critically important it is to *let* such thoughts go away, rather than trying to *make* them disappear. The harder you try to shove obsessions out the door, I was told, the more they're going to come back in through a window. That's why compulsive rituals and other acts of desperate distraction never work for very long. The real key to managing obsessive thoughts is not to block them, but to weaken them to the point where they can be tuned out. So one of the biggest lessons of CBT was that I should open the door, let the thoughts in, and live my life—trusting that the thoughts would get bored and stop visiting so often once my strategy became clear and consistently implemented.

I was learning fast, and I was mentally kicking myself for being so petulant about trying CBT in the first place. Now that I had given it a shot, I had to concede that it was working. The relief I experienced as my symptoms began to subside remains an unparalleled feeling. My mind had been enslaved to OCD for so long that I had almost forgotten what freedom felt like, but that just made it all the sweeter.

Looking East for Inspiration

The combination of CBT and medication was beginning to make a real dent in my symptoms. I decided to make the most of treatment by doing all I could on my own to calm my mind and quell my fears. As it happens, two students in my dorm were into martial arts. One practiced tae kwon do, and the other, ninjitsu. I soon learned that two members of the dorm staff also were highly trained martial artists. Between them, they had considerable experience in karate, jujitsu, and judo.

During gym class—one of my least favorite activities on the planet—I expressed an interest in learning martial arts, too. I was told that formally teaching a student at a therapeutic boarding school the art of combat, no matter how innocuous or even therapeutic the intention, was strictly forbidden. On the other hand, there wasn't anything to say that information about martial arts couldn't be worked into casual conversation. And so began my study of karate with a dorm staff member.

The first thing my newfound sensei, or teacher, taught me was that I needed to understand and come to peace with my "center" before I could hope to gain much from martial arts. This sounded a bit hokey, and I was skeptical. I had been under the impression that I could become a tough and brilliant master fighter without taking time to learn the discipline and philosophy that supported the fighting skills. It wasn't long, though, before I came to appreciate the wisdom of taking a mind-body approach.

The first few months were spent on learning breathing techniques. I have a very short attention span, so the idea of sitting still and focusing purely on the inflow and outflow of air was none too appealing to me. But I respected my karate teacher and accepted that he knew what he was doing, so I gave it a try. This type of breathing exercise is actually a form of meditation, because it involves focusing the mind intently on a particular thing or activity—in this case, the act of breathing in and out. It's an effective way of calming the mind, relaxing the body, and reducing stress.

It took a few attempts to get the hang of meditation. The first time I tried it, I looked up at my dorm staffer turned karate teacher turned best friend and told him that I couldn't do it. There were too many distracting thoughts in my head, I explained, and I would never be able to focus on something as pure and peaceful as breathing. To my surprise, he smiled and told me this was a good sign.

My teacher explained that when a distracting thought enters your mind during meditation, this isn't something to fight. Instead, you simply acknowledge the thought, understand why it is there, and dismiss it passively, allowing it to move unimpeded through your thought processes and be on its way.

Rather than fighting entering thoughts, I was taught to greet them in a noncombative way

Rather than fighting entering thoughts, I was taught to greet them in a noncombative way during meditation.

during meditation. The parallels to CBT were obvious. In CBT, I was taught not to fight obsessive thoughts, which would only intensify them. Instead, I was learning to notice such thoughts, see them for the absurdities they were, and let them fade away on their own as they lost their power.

At first, I found it exceedingly difficult to practice passive disregard during meditation. But once I began to master the meditative attitude, I realized that it was one of the best things I had stumbled across in quite some time. Suddenly, I wasn't terrified; I was aware. I learned to let go of the anger and frustration that had been dragging me down. It was *my* baggage, after all, and it dawned on me that I didn't have to continue carrying it around if I didn't want to.

After a few months, I moved on to studying the physical practice of karate. I learned basic defensive and offensive postures. I practiced hitting correctly and aligning my body and mind to focus my energy into a single fluid action. For once, I felt my body working with itself, not against itself.

I had been very angry about the fact that my life was consumed by obsessions and compulsions I wanted no part of. I sometimes had episodes of extreme rage to the point of tears. But over time, thanks largely to CBT and meditation, I came to peace with the pain that had been bottled up inside.

I turned rage into insight and muscle, and I shed the sense of helplessness that had been eating me up inside. The lessons I learned back then have carried me through many subsequent experiences: quitting smoking, applying to college, even graduating at the top of my college class. I learned to control myself, not let OCD control me. And as my mind slipped free of its shackles, I came to see that life is not meant to be lived in fear, but in awe of all the amazing and bizarre things we have the privilege to see. Liberation is one of the greatest feelings in the world.

The Big Picture

I tried several different treatments with several different doctors and therapists before I found the best combination for me. This is a common experience. OCD is a complex problem that doesn't have a one-size-fits-all solution. Instead, it requires an individualized approach. If you're still searching for the right approach for you, try not to be discouraged. One thing I've realized in hindsight is that even the failures were useful. By learning what didn't work for me, my treatment providers and I were able to narrow down the options and find what did.

OCD is a brain disorder, so the most effective treatments are ones that change how the brain works. Surprisingly, this applies to both medication and CBT. Recent research suggests that both types of treatment produce similar changes in brain function. Specifically, after several weeks of therapy with either an SSRI medication or CBT, studies have shown that areas of the brain that tend to be hyperactive in OCD return to a more normal level of activity. The implication is clear: Although medication and CBT look like very different approaches on the outside, they actually may work through similar mechanisms inside the brain.

Both CBT and medication can be helpful. Dr. Martin Franklin, the scientific author of this book, was one of a team of researchers who studied the effectiveness of CBT, SSRI medication, or a combination of both for treating OCD in children and teenagers. The study was a randomized controlled trial (see the box on the following page) that included 112

What's a Randomized Controlled Trial?

If you read much about clinical research, you're bound to come across the term "randomized controlled trial." This type of study is "randomized" because participants are randomly divided into treatment and control groups. Randomization helps ensure that the groups are as comparable as possible. It's "controlled" because there is a control group for comparison's sake. This group typically receives a dummy pill (placebo), a nonspecific psychotherapy, or simply standard care without any extra treatment added. The big plus to this study design is that it lets researchers determine which changes in the treatment group over time are due to the treatment itself.

young people at three university treatment centers. All three treatments were more effective at reducing symptoms than a placebo, a sugar pill that looks like the real medication but doesn't contain an active ingredient.

Taken together, the results from the three treatment centers showed that young people did better on a combination of CBT and an SSRI than on either treatment alone. However, for those treated at the University of Pennsylvania, CBT alone worked as well as the combined treatment. The moral: The way therapists provide CBT is a big factor in determining how well it works.

Whether you try CBT, an SSRI, or both, it usually takes a few weeks for the effects to start kicking in. It's important to give any treatment a fair trial before concluding that it isn't working. That generally means sticking with it for at least ten weeks. If you're concerned that you aren't improving as much or as quickly as you had

It's important to give any treatment a fair trial before concluding that it isn't working.

expected, talk to your doctor or therapist. Don't just stop the treatment, as that may lead to an increase in symptoms.

What Form of CBT Is Most Effective?

Based on research, the first-choice treatment for teens with OCD is usually either CBT combined with an SSRI medication or CBT alone. One particular form of CBT, known as exposure and response prevention (EX/RP), has proved to be especially effective. It has two main components: *exposure* to the situations that trigger obsessive thoughts and *prevention* of the compulsive rituals that are the person's usual response. When someone repeatedly faces his or her fears without falling back on compulsions, the anxiety that's evoked starts to lessen over time.

The first step in EX/RP is to develop a hierarchy of feared situations, from those that produce the least anxiety to those that produce the most. The person starts by confronting a fairly low-anxiety situation. Once this challenge has been met, the person moves step by step up the hierarchy, tackling more and more difficult situations.

In Vivo Exposure

The exposure part of EX/RP can take place either in real life or in the person's imagination. In vivo exposure is the real-life kind. It involves coming into contact with the actual anxiety-provoking situation. For instance, an obsessive cleaner might be asked to run his or her hands through a tub of dirt or rummage through a trashcan, while an obsessive counter might be asked to tap the table or flip the light switch an "unlucky" 13 times.

One teaching technique is modeling, in which the therapist demonstrates exposure. At first, the person might simply watch as the therapist comes into contact with the feared situation without resorting to any rituals. Later, the person might be asked to follow the therapist's example of how to respond (or not respond) in these situations.

IMAGINED EXPOSURE

Imagined exposure involves coming into contact with an anxiety-provoking situation through mental imagery. It's used when real-life exposure would be impractical or impossible—for example, when a person has intrusive images of burning in hell because a blasphemous thought was allowed to go un-challenged. The therapist describes the feared scene using a lot of sensory detail until the person has a clear picture of it in mind. Then the therapist continues with the worst-case sce-nario, detailing the negative consequences that the person fears will occur.

Let's say someone with a checking obsession fears that a burglar will break into his home because he hasn't checked the doors to make sure they're locked. The therapist might graphically describe a scene in which this happens. Rather than trying to squelch the anxiety that's aroused, the person lets himself experience the feeling. As the scene is described over and over, it starts to lose some of its power, and the anxiety begins to fade. When the person can imagine this scene without growing more anxious, the therapist moves on to the next scenario.

RESPONSE PREVENTION

Whether the exposure takes place in the real world or the mind's eye, response prevention always occurs along with it. This just means that the person refrains from acting out—or imagining acting out—compulsive rituals in response. Al-though the therapist is there to offer guidance and support, the restraint needed to prevent rituals is always self-imposed. It's never forced upon anyone.

For instance, let's say a compulsive hand-washer worries that touching "germy" doorknobs will make her sick. Even if she touches doorknobs every day and never becomes ill as a result, she might tell herself it's only because she washed her hands so thoroughly afterward. In EX/RP, this person would not only touch doorknobs, but also refrain from washing her hands for several hours afterward. Over time, when she didn't get sick, she would come to realize that her old belief about the necessity of constant washing wasn't true. The power of doorknobs to evoke anxiety would begin to fade.

EX/RP IN ACTION

While exposure and response prevention are described separately above, they actually occur at the same time and work together in therapy. The overarching goal of EX/RP is to turn into your fear rather than away from it—adding the gruesome details where needed and keeping your mind focused on the anxious thoughts. At the same time, you make a conscious effort not to distract yourself from the thoughts and not to provide yourself with subtle reassurance in the form of mental rituals, for example, by silently saying "I would never do that" during an imagined exposure that relates to harming a loved one.

Even after the exposure session ends, response prevention continues. This is important to keep from undoing some of the good that was done during the session. So once you walk out the door of your therapist's office, you still make an effort not to go out and engage in ritualistic behavior.

WHAT TO EXPECT FROM EX/RP

EX/RP isn't an easy fix. It requires taking an active role in your own treatment and confronting high-anxiety situations head-on.

In the short run, this can lead to a temporary increase in anxiety. In the long run, however, it can save you enormous suffering by giving you effective tools for managing OCD.

In general, long exposures pack more punch than brief ones. The idea is to wait until your anxiety level peaks and then starts to come back down, and that can take some time. Therefore, exposure sessions with your therapist usually last at least 45 minutes and sometimes longer. The frequency of sessions depends partly upon how severe your symptoms are. For very severe symptoms, frequent or even daily sessions might be advised at first. For more moderate symptoms, weekly sessions might be enough.

Your therapist can guide you through EX/RP, but it's up to you to do the work. Response avoidance needs to be practiced not only in the therapist's office but also at home between visits. Family members and friends can act as support persons, but neither your therapist nor your supporters will force you to do anything against your will. It's your job to give response avoidance your best effort. The more effort you put in, the more benefit you'll get out of the treatment.

> It's your job to give response avoidance your best effort.

A potential drawback to EX/RP is that optimal results might depend on finding an experienced cognitive-behavioral therapist. Unfortunately, in many parts of the country, such therapists are few and far between. Your family doctor, psychiatrist, or psychologist may be able to recommend a CBT specialist. Also, the Anxiety Disorders Association of America (www.adaa. org), Obsessive-Compulsive Foundation (www.ocfoundation. org), and Association for Behavioral and Cognitive Therapies (www.abct.org) offer searchable online directories of treatment providers.

A Booster Shot of Therapy

CBT is an effective set of tools, but like any tools, they can get a little rusty with time. For me, that time came while I was at college. My symptoms worsened until they were getting in the way of my schoolwork and life in general. It took me about six weeks to finally admit that I wasn't in control anymore.

I talked to my therapist at the college health center, and he and I agreed that it was probably a good idea to call Dr. C., my cognitive-behavioral therapist, and schedule an appointment. At first, I felt as if I had failed, but Dr. C. assured me that many people with OCD need occasional sessions after the intensive therapy is over to make sure they keep using the tools properly and don't fall back into the same old habits.

In my case, I had started allowing myself a small amount of time each day for rituals, reasoning that it was harmless. But with my guard down, those few minutes soon mushroomed into hours. A few booster sessions with Dr. C. helped me take charge of my life again. I also learned to set boundaries with myself and stick to them. Since then, I've come to accept that keeping myself as healthy as possible is a lifelong job, and a tune-up now and then helps maintain my progress.

One major advantage of all CBT approaches, including EX/RP, is that they teach you anxiety management skills you can use for the rest of your life. Studies have shown that many people are still feeling better months or years after the conclusion of therapy. The same typically isn't true of medication. Some research suggests that the benefits of medication may recede soon after people stop taking their medicine. However, more recent studies suggest that the benefits might be longer lasting if the medication is tapered off slowly.

COGNITIVE FORMS OF CBT

EX/RP is the best-studied type of psychotherapy for OCD in young people. However, more purely cognitive forms of CBT also have proved helpful for adults with the disorder. These approaches are based on the assumption that people with OCD have irrational beliefs along with their obsessions. Examples of such beliefs include:

- Thinking about performing an action is the same as doing it.
- Not trying to prevent harm is the same as causing the harm.
- It's necessary to be vigilant all the time to prevent disasters.

Everyone has unwanted thoughts from time to time. According to one theory, people with OCD overreact to these thoughts, seeing them as potentially harmful and feeling personally responsible for the bad things that might occur afterward. This type of thinking naturally produces a lot of anxiety, and compulsions are a vain attempt to keep the anxiety at bay. Cognitive therapies try to get to the heart of the disorder by helping people recognize and challenge their irrational beliefs.

ACCEPTANCE AND COMMITMENT THERAPY

Acceptance and commitment therapy (ACT; pronounced "act" rather than spelled out) is a new offshoot of CBT. It combines acceptance of inner experience and commitment to behavior change with mindfulness, a form of meditation that involves fully focusing attention on whatever is being experienced here and now without judging or reacting to it. ACT is an interesting idea that closely resembles the mixture of CBT and meditation that worked so well for me. But so far, only limited research has been done on ACT, so it's impossible to say yet whether it has widespread potential as a treatment for OCD.

What Types of Medication Are Helpful?

If CBT alone doesn't provide enough relief, the combination of CBT and medication may. And if the first combination you try doesn't do the job, there are several options. Your treatment provider may change to more intensive CBT, adjust the medication dosage, switch to a different medication, or add a second medication. It's all a matter of mixing and matching treatments to find the best overall strategy for you. While CBT is the cornerstone of OCD treatment, medication also has an important role to play.

The combination of medicine and CBT may be especially helpful for people with moderate to severe symptoms. It also may be beneficial for those who have both OCD and certain other disorders that respond well to medication, such as another anxiety disorder or depression. On the other hand, in a recent study, Dr. Franklin and his colleagues found that young people with both OCD and a tic disorder were helped by CBT but not by medication alone.

Fortunately, more research has been done on medication therapy for OCD than for any other anxiety disorder. There's good evidence for the effectiveness of two types of medication: SSRIs and an older type of antidepressant called clomipramine (Anafranil).

SELECTIVE SEROTONIN REUPTAKE INHIBITORS:
- citalopram (Celexa)
- escitalopram (Lexapro)
- fluoxetine (Prozac)
- fluvoxamine (Luvox)
- paroxetine (Paxil)
- sertraline (Zoloft)

SSRIs are classified as antidepressants, but they're also widely used to treat anxiety disorders. In the brain, SSRIs increase the concentration and activity of serotonin, a chemical that seems to play a central role in OCD. Large, well-controlled studies have shown that three SSRIs—fluoxetine, fluvoxamine, and sertraline—are effective for treating children and teens with OCD. All three of these drugs have been approved by the U.S. Food and Drug Administration (FDA) for that purpose.

Possible side effects include upset stomach, decreased appetite, headache, tiredness, and sexual problems. Mild side effects often go away on their own in a few days. If the side effects are more severe, though, your doctor might be able to change your dosage or medication. In addition, some people who take antidepressants develop increased anxiety, panic attacks, trouble sleeping, irritability, hostility, impulsiveness, agitation, or restlessness. It's thought that those who develop these symptoms soon after starting an antidepressant may be at increased risk for suicidal thoughts. If you notice these symptoms, be sure to *let your doctor know right away.*

Clomipramine (Anafranil)

Clomipramine belongs to an older group of antidepressants. Like SSRIs, this drug affects the concentration and activity of serotonin in the brain. However, it also has several other chemical effects inside the body that may be unwanted. It was the first medication to be systematically studied in children and teens with OCD. Studies found it effective, and it received FDA approval as an OCD treatment for young people.

But since clomipramine is more likely to cause troublesome side effects than SSRIs, it usually isn't a first-choice treatment. Possible side effects include drowsiness, dizziness, dry mouth, upset stomach, constipation, sexual problems, changes in weight or appetite, bladder problems, shakiness, and increased heart rate. The FDA warning about the risk of suicidal thoughts applies to clomipramine, too.

WHAT TO EXPECT FROM MEDICATION

For CBT to work, you really need to focus on therapy, but that's very difficult to do when obsessive thoughts are monopolizing your mind. Medication may suppress symptoms enough to make it easier to concentrate—one reason the combination of CBT and medication is so powerful.

Different people respond differently to the same drug based on factors such as age, sex, weight, body chemistry, and overall health. Finding the best medication and dosage for you may take some trial and error. Never just stop taking your medicine without talking to your doctor first, though, since stopping too abruptly may lead to unpleasant withdrawal symptoms.

Finding the best medication and dosage for you may take some trial and error.

Once you find an antidepressant that helps, you'll usually keep taking it for at least 6 to 12 months and sometimes longer.

One drawback to medication is the possibility of side effects. Be sure to consult your doctor about any new symptoms that develop soon after you start a new medication. However, the risk of side effects must be balanced against the consequences of letting OCD go untreated. Left unchecked, OCD can cause substantial suffering and make it almost impossible to do the things you want to do. Medication may reduce the distress and decrease the day-to-day problems, helping you reclaim your life.

How Can I Pay for Treatment?

Finding treatment is one thing. Paying for it can be quite another. Even if you or your parents have health insurance, the coverage for mental health care often isn't as extensive as that for other medical services. Call the customer service number for your insurance plan to find out what's covered and what isn't. Here are some questions to ask:

- Do I need a referral from my family doctor before seeing a psychiatrist or therapist?
- Must I choose my psychiatrist or therapist from a network of approved providers?
- How much will my deductible and co-payment be? The deductible is the amount of health care costs that you or your parents must pay out-of-pocket each year before health insurance starts paying. Once insurance kicks in, it often only pays part of the cost for covered services. The co-payment is the portion of the costs that you or your parents are responsible for paying.
- Is there a limit on the number of visits to a treatment provider or days in a treatment facility that insurance will cover?
- Is there a yearly or lifetime cap on the total amount that insurance will pay for mental health services?

Most health insurance plans will only cover services that satisfy the standard for "medical necessity," which means the services are deemed medically appropriate and necessary to meet your health care needs. If you're ever denied coverage for a service that your treatment provider thinks you need, ask your insurance company about the procedure for appealing the decision. Mental Health America, a nonprofit organization, also offers easy-to-understand pointers on this topic. Visit www.mentalhealthamerica.net, and search for "treatment denials."

If you don't have private insurance, you still might qualify for coverage through Medicaid or the State Child Health Insurance Program (SCHIP), two government programs that provide medical and mental health care to those who meet eligibility criteria. Medicaid provides health insurance to eligible low-income and disabled individuals, while SCHIP provides health insurance for the children in certain lower-income families who aren't eligible for Medicaid. Program specifics vary from state to state. To find out exactly what your state offers, start with GovBenefits.gov (800-333–4636, www.govbenefits.gov). If you're 18 or younger, also check out Insure Kids Now! (877-543–7669, www.insurekidsnow.gov).

Many people are caught in a gray area. They don't have adequate coverage under private insurance, but they also don't qualify for government programs. If that's your situation, ask whether your treatment provider offers reduced fees or a payment plan. Community mental health centers are another option. They provide a wide range of mental health services regardless of ability to pay. Fees are set on a sliding scale based on your or your parents' income and the cost of services. Also, if you're having trouble affording your medication, many pharmaceutical companies offer assistance programs to people with financial needs. For more details, contact the Partnership for Prescription Assistance (888-477–2669, www.pparx.org).

Finally, if you have the opportunity, you might want to consider volunteering to take part in a clinical trial that's studying treatments for OCD. By participating, you may gain access to high-quality care for free. You'll be fully informed about potential risks and benefits before you sign up. If you're a minor, a parent or guardian will need to give consent. To learn more about clinical trials and search for ones that are currently seeking volunteers in your area, check out the listings maintained by the National Library of Medicine (www. clinicaltrials.gov).

Which Self-Help Strategies Are Useful?

OCD is a serious illness that needs professional care. Once you've started psychotherapy and/or medication, though, there are things you can do for yourself to feel better and make the most of treatment. For me, meditation and karate were invaluable. Here are some general pointers that may help you help yourself:

- Stick with your treatment plan. At times, you may feel uncomfortable or impatient, but don't give up. Persistence pays off, as my own experience shows.
- Consider joining a support group. This is a group of people with a common problem who get together to share emotional support, practical advice, and sometimes educational resources. Just meeting other people who are struggling with some of the same challenges as you are can be tremendously reassuring. If nothing else, it lets you know that you're not in this battle alone. The Obsessive-Compulsive Foundation (www.ocfoundation. org) and Anxiety Disorders Association of America (www.adaa.org) both offer online lists of support groups around the country.
- Enlist the help of loved ones. Family members and friends can be peerless sources of support and encouragement when you hit potholes in the road to recovery.

- Get regular physical activity. Results from a small study in adults suggest that regular aerobic exercise might help reduce OCD symptoms. Aerobic exercise is the kind that uses the large muscles of the arms and legs and speeds up your heart rate for a sustained period. Examples include jogging, brisk walking, cycling, swimming laps, inline skating, and cross-country skiing. Of course, exercise has many other benefits, too. The list includes increasing self-esteem, fighting depression, toning muscles, building strong bones, and helping maintain a healthy weight.

> Results from a small study in adults suggest that regular aerobic exercise might help reduce OCD symptoms.

- Educate yourself about OCD. The more you know about your illness, the better prepared you'll be to maximize the benefits of treatment. You'll also be ready to cope with symptoms as soon as they arise and get help promptly when you need it.
- Avoid seeking chemical solutions. Alcohol and drug abuse just create new problems without solving any of the old ones. Chapter 5 has more information on this topic.

What's the Least I Need to Know?

Effective treatments for OCD are available. But even with successful treatment, OCD is usually a long-lasting disorder. While the symptoms may get much better, they might not go away completely. Any symptoms that remain may come and go for years. At times, they might disappear completely, only

The Write Stuff

At one point, I was encouraged by my doctor to start a journal. The idea was to keep a log of triggers and fears to discuss in therapy. However, I found that the benefits of writing about what was happening in my life went far beyond just jogging my memory. I was spending a lot of time in my head terrified of the next catastrophe, no matter how farfetched or irrational it might seem. It was very hard to hold those fears up for scrutiny by another person. In fact, I find myself still embarrassed to admit some of my old fears, even the ones that are long since under control.

But "talking" to my personal journal was a totally different matter. I learned to share my deepest thoughts and feelings there without holding back. It's amazing what you can express on paper—things that are much more difficult to say out loud. Eventually, I became comfortable sharing some of these written musings with my therapist. And that, in turn, made it easier to talk about them. Thanks to my journal, I became better able to convey what I was going through in a clear, cohesive manner.

My love affair with writing was born out of this. As you might expect, that's why this book exists. It turns out that I really was writing for my life.

to return when you're under stress. For this reason, it's best to think of managing OCD as a long-term undertaking—not something you do once and then forget about.

The good news is that once you've mastered some basic techniques for resisting OCD behaviors, you can use them over and over. CBT, either alone or combined with medication, teaches you lifelong skills that can help you not only feel better now, but also maintain your improvement in the future.

Chapter Five

Rituals, Routines, and Recovery: Living With OCD

My Story

It was during my junior year of high school that I experienced the most horrific and terrifying obsessions. These intrusive thoughts included images that superimposed themselves upon the world around me like an acetate overlay. For instance, in the middle of a conversation with my best friend, Corrine, I would suddenly see myself burying a hatchet into her chest. It was the most terrifying thing I could think of, since I loved Corrine (and still do to this day). Yet this sort of image kept coming back at random times, and when it did, it left me shaking.

I also developed a fear that if I didn't tell my therapist every single thing I had done the entire day, it would turn out that I had omitted the part where I killed someone and left the body in the woods. To my knowledge, I've never actually killed anyone, and I've certainly never left a dead body in the woods. But the thought kept returning. This was my OCD telling me that I had done something I found morally reprehensible.

Sometimes in the middle of a therapy session, I would tell my therapist that I was afraid I was going to hit him or do him bodily harm in some other way. I expected him to be horrified and offended, but he explained that this is a very common belief among people being treated for OCD. If the violent thoughts truly are due to OCD, there's very little chance that they'll turn into real acts of violence. On the other hand, they could easily give rise to compulsive rituals. In my case, I would exhaustively confess every tiny wrongdoing, often while sitting on my hands to make sure I didn't do something even more terrible.

There were also occasions when I mentally saw myself rape or molest someone, and the images scared the hell out of me. When I told my therapist about these intrusive thoughts, I started to shake. Over and over, I said that I didn't think I had done it, but what if I had? What if I were a super-villainous serial rapist who had figured out how to elude the police and the FBI where others had failed? I was terrified that I was leading a double life—sweet on the outside but with a personality on the inside that made Jack the Ripper look like a Boy Scout.

Over and over, I said that I didn't think I had done it, but what if I had?

Staring Down OCD

Dr. C., my cognitive-behavioral therapist, has degrees in several fields, one of which is divinity. This made me wonder if perhaps I might be confessing my sins rather than explaining my obsessions to him. And though I feared that I possibly could be sort of a serial killer, over time, I came to accept Dr. C.'s assurances that I was not. At first, I was a little skeptical, but I trusted the man. Here was someone who not only was a doctor who healed people mentally and emotionally, but also had a connection to God. I believed this connection would require him to drive a stake through my heart if he deemed me to be anywhere near as evil as I had previously assumed myself to be.

Dr. C. asked whether I enjoyed the thoughts about acting violently—a very straightforward question I probably should have asked myself long before. My immediate reaction was that *of course* I didn't. The thoughts were sometimes so terrible that I lost sleep and had to be sedated for panic-induced shortness of breath and palpitations. Then Dr. C. asked another really good question that should have been obvious: Was it likely that I would be an evil murderer if the mere thought of violence was so distressing to me? Finally, Dr. C. asked whether I had been visited by the police. I told him I hadn't. I realized right then that he was showing me how completely illogical it was to believe that the horrible images were true.

The next thing we did was extremely unnerving. Dr. C. asked me to free associate words related to all manner of violent acts, particularly the ones I found most abhorrent and unforgivable, such as molestation, rape, and murder. I went through a thesaurus' worth of words, then continued into words that had been causing me to think of these violent thoughts. Dr. C. wrote it all down on his scratchpad. When he was finished, he asked if it was okay for him to show me what he had written. I was surprised that the request scared me so deeply.

On the page were words so vile and disturbing that they went against everything I held sacred and important. The acts named there were far removed from what I believed to be morally correct and not even in the vicinity of anything I would ever do. As I stared at the words, images flashed through my mind like a rapid-fire slide show of the most horrible scenes I could imagine. I was terrified. This, Dr. C. told me, was the first step toward facing down my OCD.

I just wanted to puke on the rug. I felt compelled to call everyone who was an authority figure in my life and ask if they could check in their area to make sure I hadn't done anything bad or hurt anyone. I also had a strong urge to call the police myself to make sure there weren't any missing person reports or crime scenes that matched the images in my head. But I didn't do these things. Instead, I just sat there and sweated it out, drenching my shirt with salty tears and sweat. In short, I went through the basic steps of EX/RP—exposure plus response prevention.

I felt very empowered knowing that the things I most feared about myself were extremely unlikely and, in some cases, utterly impossible. Yet the words didn't lose their anxiety-provoking ability overnight. When the therapy session ended, I took the list with me and tucked it away, feeling almost as if I needed a biohazard bag to contain it. Over repeated exposures, though, I came to know the words intimately. I also exposed myself to violent media and challenged myself by asking if I could even remotely be the sort of person who did such terrible things.

> *I felt very empowered knowing that the things I most feared about myself were extremely unlikely*

On the plus side, I got the privilege of viewing some really nasty horror movies that the other kids weren't allowed to watch at school. Some of the kids were even jealous of my therapy.

Life Beyond High School

Before I found EX/RP, I was struggling—not only with the symptoms of OCD itself, but also with related problems. As I later discovered, having other psychological and behavioral problems in addition to OCD is quite common. In my case, I found myself using drugs to make the pain go away, and I smoked cigarettes, too, in a sarcastic approach to casual and gradual suicide. At various times, I also had to contend with panic attacks, depression, and recurring tics.

After I began getting my symptoms under control with effective treatment, I made a lot of progress. I quit smoking, graduated from high school with honors, and became more comfortable with who I was. It wasn't an overnight miracle cure, however, and the comfort had its limits. Although the symptoms became milder and more manageable, they didn't disappear.

In college, I started allowing obsessions and rituals back into my life like unwanted houseguests who wouldn't go away. My schedule of college activities dictated that I have a routine every day, and I followed it precisely, even compulsively. I spent most of my college career using several alarm clocks at once, setting them to go off at different times in a sequence that wasn't predictable. I also made sure each clock was at least five feet away from my bed so that I wouldn't be able to just hit the snooze button and go back to sleep. Yet I still lost a lot of sleep to perpetual anxiety over the possibility of missing a single minute of class.

The stress of not getting enough sleep combined with the transition to college life was tough on me. Almost all teenagers yearn for greater freedom. But suddenly being plopped into a situation with very few restrictions after the structure of a therapeutic boarding school was harder than I had expected. Of course, I wasn't alone in that feeling. Many college freshmen are shocked to discover that there is such a thing as having too much freedom. When OCD symptoms are added to the mix, however, the pressure can feel overwhelming.

Hoarding 101

College students aren't known for their tidiness, so when you live in the basement of a dorm the way I did, dirt is unavoidable. I resigned myself to the knowledge that I was constantly surrounded by germs and there was nothing I could do about it. In that environment, I made great strides toward overcoming my contamination fears, but new problems with hoarding cropped up.

In college, it's easy to become a packrat. I got into the habit of throwing things onto my desk in between classes and social activities. Later I would stuff everything into a drawer or shove it out of sight. For most students, this might lead to nothing worse than a messy room. But for me, it triggered a tendency toward compulsive hoarding.

During my first year of college, like many people, I went through a sort of reinvention of self that included refining how I dressed. I bought a new wardrobe, but still I kept all the clothing I no longer wore. I would estimate that I used up to 75% of my closet space to store clothes that didn't fit me or that I didn't like. The fear was that, if I did throw them away, I would be losing something of myself. Although many people feel that way about a certain blanket or favorite old sweater, I felt that way about everything I owned. I could not, to the point of absurdity, part with anything. More to the point, I had to keep it all on hand.

In addition to clothes, I also kept all kinds of old computer equipment in case I ever needed it—which meant I planned to save it for eternity. As a technician building computers out of old junk parts, my job was to extract what I needed from machines that still ran well and scrap the rest. Instead, my office in the engineering building began to overflow with old intake fans, floppy discs, and cables. Whenever forced to justify keeping these things, I became quite defensive, creating elaborate scenarios in which I might need a five-inch floppy drive in the future despite the fact that they had been obsolete for nearly two decades. I sometimes felt the overwhelming sense that, if I didn't have the parts on hand, I would one day be unprepared for a catastrophe.

Then there were the mounds of paper. I remember looking around my dorm room one day and thinking that it was gradually and inexplicably shrinking. When I sifted through my drawers later that night, a pile of receipts from the bookstore, drugstore, and several dozen other stores fell onto the floor. Pulling out a big trunk from underneath my bed, I found more receipts inside.

On my bookshelf, there was a binder with several pocket folders designed to store receipts and record transactions. Its intended purpose was to help me organize my finances. But as noble as that goal was, it really wasn't the underlying motive. The true driving force was an unexplained fear that one of these days I would find myself in dire need of proof

The problem was that I was keeping the receipts indefinitely for every single item I paid for.

that I had paid for some random item. I also worried that my personal information might leak out if I didn't keep a tight lid on it, and that meant not casually tossing out receipts. The problem was that I was keeping the receipts indefinitely for every single item I paid for.

I had such limited space to begin with that I wasn't able to rationalize the hoarding for long. I couldn't afford to keep collecting extraneous trash if I didn't want to be evicted for health reasons. Besides, I was starting to lose my current homework in the piles of homework from long ago.

Yet I reasoned that I could never be absolutely sure that a piece of paper or scrap of information was no longer useful. I kept all my old assignment sheets, telling myself that one day the professors could somehow lose all of my work and I would have to reproduce it. Many of the papers were either expired assignments turned in long ago or drafts of essays that had been long since revised, so part of me realized that they were unlikely to be of use, but the very idea of parting with them was still terrifying.

Cleaning Up My Act

I realized it was time to do a serious intervention with myself—to clean out the drawers, clear off the shelves, and sort through my trunk and closet. By a stroke of good fortune, Radio Shack was having a sale on paper shredders—the heavy-duty, cross-cut kind. I bought one of those bad boys and made a pile of papers to get rid of. Then I promptly panicked and had to run outside for a deep breath.

By coaxing a friend to come back inside with me, I finally was able to start the destruction of many pounds of unwanted paper under the guise of showing off a new toy. Never underestimate the young male's desire to demonstrate his masculinity by destroying stuff. The allure of grinding gears wasn't lost on my friends, and I eventually had what I called a shredding party. Seven shopping bags later, you could see dust clouding in the room from the gears tearing away at all that paper. I haven't lived without a shredder since then.

Next I decided to take on the old, unworn clothes. First I took some big brown paper bags and started to stuff them with old jackets. Then I began filling garbage bags with designer skater clothing. When I donated the bags to Goodwill afterward, I realized that I had just managed to not only do an exposure for myself, but also help others who were less fortunate in the process—a really worthwhile return on my investment of time, energy, and effort.

Finally, I tackled the old computer equipment I had been saving for the proverbial rainy day that never came. I was (and still am) heavily into computers and technology, so there was a lot of it. I took out the old components and stripped them down to their base level. Then I dusted them, repainted a couple, installed upgraded parts, and made whole computers out of the garbage that had been invading my personal space. I donated the computers to a local nonprofit organization that provides services and support to survivors of domestic abuse. So in another exposure, I not only sharpened my computer repair skills, but also made new computers for people who really needed them. Now that's something to feel doubly good about.

The Big Picture

OCD can be simultaneously your worst enemy and your best friend. Every time I overcame obsessive-compulsive thoughts and behavior, I learned more about myself and took greater charge of my life. As a result, I'm of the sincerely peculiar opinion that some good has come from my illness. I can't honestly say that I'm grateful for OCD, but I do think it has made me a stronger, better person.

Comorbidity—in other words, the coexistence of two or more disorders in the same person—just adds to the challenge. Mental health professionals use strict criteria to define different disorders for purposes of diagnosis, treatment, and research. This creates the illusion of neat, orderly categories. But real life

Uncluttering Your Life

Being a run-of-the-mill packrat is one thing. But being a truly compulsive hoarder is quite another. Hoarding—the excessive collection of items with little or no apparent value—is a serious problem that needs professional treatment. In addition to following your treatment plan, these steps can help you find your way out of the clutter:

- Learn more about the problem. The Obsessive-Compulsive Foundation's Compulsive Hoarding website (www.ocfoundation. org/hoarding) is a good starting place.
- Get out and socialize. If you're embarrassed to invite visitors over, meet your friends at their homes or in public places.
- Keep up your hygiene. It can be hard to dust tabletops, vacuum floors, or find clean clothes amid piles of stuff, but don't let that stop you.
- Donate or recycle unneeded items. These alternatives to simply throwing things out let you help others while you help yourself.
- Consider buying a shredder if you tend to hoard printed matter. Open your mail next to the shredder, and keep only what's essential.
- Take the same approach to e-mail—save only what you really need, and delete the rest. Create an efficient, workable filing system for the e-mails you save.

is much messier than that, and many teens have symptoms of more than one condition.

As I've mentioned, I faced several challenges—including depression, substance abuse, and a tic disorder—in addition to OCD. I learned that it was important to address *all* of them. Otherwise, the symptoms tended to feed each other and keep the problems going. It's hard to concentrate on OCD in therapy, for instance, when your motivation is sapped by depression or your ability to think clearly is undermined by drugs. That's one reason treatment needs to be individualized. You're one of a kind, and your exact mix of symptoms and conditions is unique, too.

All Hallows' Eve

I've had trouble with the holidays as far back as I can remember. It's not that I don't like them, but the collective unease of people around me added to the stress of a significant day makes for anxiety. Somehow it seems that intrusive thoughts are lent more credence merely because of a particular day on the calendar.

Halloween is one holiday I usually don't have trouble with. But as I'm writing this passage on the morning of October 31, scrupulosity is rearing its head. Just to give you a little background, a few months ago, I found myself getting more and more depressed. I had recently graduated from college, and the world didn't seem as friendly and full of opportunity as I had been led to believe. Then out of the blue, I was offered a chance to write this book. While it was a wonderful surprise and an amazing opportunity, it also meant I had to cope with a whole new set of stresses and pressures.

I turned to a source of strength I had been neglecting of late: prayer. Ashamed that I hadn't been showing gratitude to a higher power the way I had been taught in addiction recovery, I started to pray a little bit each day. At first, prayer was a source of comfort. Then without warning, I suddenly felt as if I needed God's permission to do anything, and I believed that I was constantly being frowned upon from on high.

Which brings me to Halloween. Tonight my girlfriend and I are throwing a costume party. The theme is Good vs. Evil, and guests are required to show up as members of one side or the other. In a way, it's the ultimate exposure, because I'll be forced to come face to face with the very things that cause me great anxiety. I've chosen to lead the Good side, which is actually very difficult to feel comfortable with.

As I was designing a flyer for the event, the thought kept returning that I was exploiting God for my own personal benefit—an act that I was convinced made me a heretic. Now that the party is almost here, I'm still uncomfortable. Yet I also believe that to have fun and raise people's spirits, and to do so with festivities and camaraderie rather than alcohol and marijuana, is a good thing. I'm determined to make this a positive experience—one more step on the journey toward recovery.

How Does Substance Abuse Affect OCD?

Technically speaking, substance abuse refers to the use of alcohol or other drugs despite negative consequences. The unwanted results can include dangerous behavior, such as driving erratically, getting into fights, having unprotected sex, or putting yourself into situations where you're at risk for sexual or physical assault. There also may be personal and social consequences, such as getting into arguments, skipping class, or developing substance-related health problems. And then there are legal issues, such as underage drinking, driving under the influence, or using illegal drugs. All in all, substance abuse can wreak havoc on your life.

Some people with OCD—myself included, at one time—turn to alcohol or other drugs in a misguided effort to relieve their distress. At first, it might seem like a quick fix. In the long run, though, it only creates a whole new set of problems to go along with the old ones. To make matters worse, alcohol or other drugs can actually trigger or worsen anxiety in certain people.

... alcohol or other drugs can actually trigger or worsen anxiety in certain people.

A common question is how addictive behavior and OCD rituals are related. You often hear drug use referred to as "compulsive." But from a scientific point of view, that's inaccurate. People who are addicted to drugs are driven to use them because it gives them temporary pleasure. (The same is true of other types of addictive behavior, such as gambling addiction.) In contrast, people with OCD are driven to repeat compulsive rituals because it gives them temporary relief from anxiety. In both cases, though, the benefit gained is short-lived. Both addictive behavior and OCD rituals make you feel worse, not better, over the long term.

If you think you might have a problem with alcohol or other drugs, reach out for help. Although many people think they can kick the problem on their own, that's very difficult to do, and having OCD just makes it harder. If you're already in treatment for OCD, be honest with your therapist or doctor about your drinking or drug use. If you're not in treatment yet, talk to a supportive adult, such as a parent, school nurse or counselor, or family doctor.

Marijuana in the OCD Brain

It's folly to think that you as an adolescent won't face the chance or the pressure to use marijuana at parties. In our culture, experimentation with drugs is often considered a normal part of growing up, for better or worse. But you should know that marijuana can negatively affect the brains of those of us with OCD, especially if we are on medication.

The use of marijuana and alcohol has been widely defended by some people with OCD, who may use it in an attempt to counter obsessions. Pot has been reported to trick people with OCD and other anxiety disorders into feeling that their OCD has disappeared, if only temporarily. However, when users come down, or "crash," the OCD symptoms return with a vengeance. The problems you were avoiding by using pot are still there, and may be fuzzier when you sober up. What's more, using marijuana and other drugs could potentially make cognitive therapy more difficult by impairing our learning and cognitive functions. The mechanisms by which marijuana affects the brain are still not well-understood, even by experts, so research is ongoing in this area.

In addition, pot and alcohol, like all drugs, interact with other psychoactive or psychiatric drugs, and not in a good way. Alcohol changes the way our blood carries nutrients, and since the liver has the job of breaking down alcohol and any drugs you're using

(continued)

(whether they're legal or illegal), its ability to process medications is compromised. Combining alcohol and psychiatric drugs, particularly SSRI medications, can be very risky and land you in the hospital. I can assure you, this is not worth the four or five hours of blundering about singing "Yankee doodle."

Aside from the awful taste of alcohol, I've found that the disorienting effects of the drug make my anxiety heighten, which is the last thing I want, as I have enough anxiety already, thank you very much. I had to make my mistakes, however, to find this out for myself. Like I said, it's not my job to be a D.A.R.E. officer and tell you what you can and can't do. I'm merely relaying facts. I was obviously your age once, and I'm still young. My friends drink and some of them smoke marijuana. I've told them that I can't take the risk and that I don't want to use these drugs, and since they're true friends, they respect that. You have nothing to prove to anyone, and you certainly aren't "weak" just because you won't take a hit or down a shot.

If you find yourself in a situation where there is alcohol or pot, let it be known to your closest friend, sometimes in advance, that you need someone to stick up for you, or even divert the attention from you. Explain why you can't, or, even better, why you don't want to use drugs. Good friends look out for each other.

How Are Tic Disorders Related to OCD?

Tics are sudden, rapid, repetitive movements or vocalizations that don't serve any useful purpose. Examples of physical tics include repeated, purposeless head jerking, grimacing, eye blinking, and tongue thrusting. Examples of vocal tics include repeated, purposeless clicking, grunting, sniffing, or coughing. Vocal tics also can include the repeated uttering of meaningless sounds or words. Up to 30% of people with OCD report having tics at some point in their lives.

From 5% to 7% of people with OCD have full-blown Tourette's syndrome, which is characterized by frequent, multiple tics. To be diagnosed with Tourette's, a person must have several physical tics and at least one vocal tic at some point in the illness, although not necessarily all at the same time. The symptoms are usually worst during the early teen years. They typically get better during the late teens or early twenties, and some people even become symptom free.

Certain tics resemble compulsive rituals. But unlike rituals, tics aren't aimed at suppressing a disturbing thought or keeping something bad from happening. Instead, they're a physical response to tension in part of the body that feels as if it needs to be released, much like the urge to sneeze.

Genes may be part of the reason why tics and OCD occur together so often. The immediate family members of people with OCD have an increased risk of developing tic disorders. The reverse is also true: Close relatives of people with Tourette's syndrome and other tic disorders have an increased risk of developing OCD. Research suggests that in some (but not all) cases, OCD and Tourette's may be different expressions of the same genetic variation.

Tics themselves often don't cause serious problems, so when people have both tics and OCD, treatment usually is focused mainly on the latter. However, CBT can help people learn not only how to manage obsessions and compulsions, but also how to cope with having frequent tics. Some therapy techniques also can help people learn how to replace one tic with another that is more socially acceptable. Collectively, these techniques often are referred to as habit reversal training. If the tics are severe, medication may be prescribed.

> CBT can help people learn not only how to manage obsessions and compulsions, but also how to cope with having frequent tics.

What Are Obsessive-Compulsive Spectrum Disorders?

The term "obsessive-compulsive spectrum disorder" is sometimes used for a group of disorders that, on the surface at least, resemble obsessions or compulsions and may respond to some of the same treatments as OCD. The whole concept of an obsessive-compulsive spectrum is still open to debate, however. The idea is that these similar-looking disorders might have the same genetic or biological roots as OCD. But although several mental and behavioral disorders are more common in people with OCD, it's unclear whether they actually share a common cause.

These are some of the conditions that have been grouped together under the obsessive-compulsive spectrum label. For whatever reason, people with OCD may have a higher-than-average risk of developing these conditions:

- Body dysmorphic disorder—A disorder in which people become so preoccupied with some imagined defect in their appearance that it causes serious distress or problems in their everyday life. People with this disorder may obsess over anything from crooked teeth or acne to knobby knees or skinny arms. They also may have some compulsions related to the way they look, such as checking themselves repeatedly in the mirror. But the obsessive thoughts and compulsive behaviors are limited to concerns about appearance. In contrast, OCD isn't limited to these concerns.
- Hypochondriasis—A disorder in which people become preoccupied with the idea that they already have a serious illness, based on their misinterpretation of harmless

body signs and sensations. Those with the disorder hold firmly to this belief, even after they've been examined by a doctor, given appropriate medical tests, and assured that everything is fine. People with hypochondriasis may have intrusive thoughts about disease, and they also may have some related compulsions, such as taking their temperature repeatedly. But the obsessions and compulsions are restricted to concerns about illness. While many people with OCD also worry about disease, they realize that their concern is overblown, and they may obsess over other things as well. In addition, people with OCD often worry more about diseases they will come down with in the future, rather than thinking that they already have a disease.

- Anorexia nervosa—An eating disorder in which people have an intense fear of gaining weight or becoming fat, even though they're underweight. People with anorexia severely restrict what they eat, often to the point of near-starvation. They worry a lot about the size and shape of their body, seeing themselves as being overweight or having some body part that's too fat despite all evidence to the contrary. They also may closely monitor their body size; for instance, by excessive weighing, repeated measuring, or frequent mirror checks. Their obsessions and compulsions are limited to concerns about body weight, however. OCD, on the other hand, isn't so limited.

- Bulimia nervosa—An eating disorder in which people binge on large amounts of food, then purge by forced vomiting or the misuse of laxatives, enemas, or diuretics (drugs that increase urination). Alternately, rather than purging, some people compensate for their eating binges by fasting or engaging in excessive exercise. As with anorexia, the person is preoccupied with concerns about body size and shape.

- Trichotillomania—A disorder in which people feel driven to pull out their own hair, leading to noticeable hair loss. The behavior isn't a true compulsion, however, because it isn't motivated by an obsession. Instead, people with trichotillomania pull out their hair in response to a rising sense of tension, which some describe as feeling like an itch. Pulling out hair often eases the tension or brings pleasure.

While there are some similarities between these disorders and OCD, there are also many differences. The overlap between the disorders isn't as large as you might think, either. People with OCD do seem to have an increased risk of developing these conditions, but the risk isn't as high as that of having OCD plus another anxiety disorder. In the same vein, people with body dysmorphic disorder or trichotillomania are more likely to have depression than OCD. For now, the jury is still out on whether an obsessive-compulsive spectrum exists.

One thing everyone agrees on, though: If you have one of these disorders in addition to OCD, it's important to get help for both conditions. Otherwise, you might not be able to make the most of your treatment.

Which Other Disorders Are Related to OCD?

Several other conditions may go hand in hand with OCD. Each presents its own particular set of challenges. Among the most common are other anxiety disorders, depression, and learning disorders.

What Is OCPD?

Obsessive-compulsive personality disorder (OCPD) and OCD sound a lot alike. In fact, they are quite different disorders. OCPD doesn't involve true obsessions or compulsions. Instead, it involves being a habitual "control freak," rule fanatic, or perfectionist to the point where this behavior pattern causes problems in daily life.

OCPD begins during the teen or young adult years. It leads to a preoccupation with control, order, and perfectionism that is long-lasting and seen in a wide range of settings. People with OCPD are often so focused on details, rules, lists, or schedules that they lose sight of what they're trying to accomplish. They may be workaholics who have trouble delegating tasks to others, or they may be perfectionists who have difficulty getting things done because of their own overly high standards. Other people might describe them as inflexible, stubborn, or overconscientious.

Like those with OCD, people with OCPD may hoard worn-out or worthless objects. However, their hoarding isn't driven by fear that a disaster will occur if they throw something out. Instead, people with OCPD just need a sense of control over their lives and environment. Given the differences between these sound-alike disorders, it's no surprise that only a small fraction of teens have both.

OTHER ANXIETY DISORDERS

Many teens with OCD have another anxiety disorder, too. As mentioned in Chapter 4, panic disorder, generalized anxiety disorder, and social anxiety disorder are especially common. Two other anxiety disorders that bear some resemblance to OCD are specific phobias and post-traumatic stress disorder (PTSD).

Specific phobias are characterized by an intense fear that is focused on a particular animal, object, activity, or situation, and that is out of proportion to any real threat. This fear leads to avoidance. People with OCD also may avoid certain things, such as dirt or "germy" objects, but their behavior is rooted in an obsession.

PTSD develops after a traumatic event. Symptoms include avoidance, emotional numbing, and increased arousal. Another common symptom is re-experiencing the trauma through vivid mental images. While OCD also can lead to disturbing images, they relate to things that might happen, not things that have already occurred.

CBT and medications are the cornerstones of treatment for all these disorders. But the specifics of treatment may vary depending on the exact nature of the problem. If you have other anxiety disorders in addition to OCD, it's important that all the disorders be addressed in your treatment plan.

DEPRESSION

In everyday conversation, people often say they're "depressed" when they feel a little blue or down in the dumps. When doctors use the term, though, they mean something more far-reaching and long-lasting. Medically speaking, depression involves being in a low mood or irritable nearly all the time, or losing interest or enjoyment in almost everything. These feelings last for at least two weeks. They're associated with other mental and physical symptoms, such as changes in eating and sleeping habits, slowed-down movements, lack of energy, feelings of worthlessness, trouble concentrating, and recurring thoughts of death. The symptoms are bad enough to cause serious distress or difficulty with day-to-day activities.

Depression often occurs side by side with OCD. For reasons that are unclear, this may be less common in teens than in adults, but the link is still strong. Overall, young people with anxiety disorders are eight times more likely than those without such disorders to suffer from depression.

CBT and antidepressants can be effective for treating not only OCD, but also depression. However, the best combination of treatments for you depends on several factors, including your personal mix of disorders and symptoms. No two individuals are exactly the same.

... the best combination of treatments for you depends on several factors, including your personal mix of disorders and symptoms.

LEARNING DISORDERS

Learning disorders are conditions that adversely affect performance at school or the ability to get along in everyday situations that call for reading, writing, or math. Such disorders appear to be relatively common in young people with OCD. When students with OCD also have learning disorders, they often have problems with handwriting, math, or written language.

Having OCD may make it harder to diagnose a learning disorder, however. That's because both conditions can interfere with speed and efficiency when doing schoolwork. It's hard to tell the difference between a student who is slowed down by OCD rituals and one who is hampered by a learning problem.

Of course, everyone has a unique learning style with stronger abilities in some areas than in others. Just because you have more trouble with math than creative writing—or vice versa—doesn't necessarily mean you have a learning disorder. Professionals look for a large gap between how well you do in school and how well you could do, given your intelligence and abilities. Identifying this type of gap requires evaluation and testing by a trained professional.

If you do have a learning disorder, the goal is to build on learning strengths while correcting and compensating for weaknesses. Special teaching methods or educational services may be helpful. And of course, if you have OCD, getting treatment helps put you in a frame of mind where you're ready to learn.

What's the Outlook for My Future?

Today I frequently give public talks about OCD, and one question I often get from teens in the audience is what the future holds. I say it's up to each person to make his or her own future. But many young adults with OCD—even those with OCD plus several coexisting conditions—go on to graduate from college, get a good job, and fall in love. I've done all those things myself now, so I know it's possible.

Looking farther down the road, you might be wondering if you'll be able to get married and raise a family, succeed at your career, buy a nice house, and achieve all the other goals you dream about. I don't have a crystal ball to answer those questions. Life doesn't come with a guarantee for *anyone*. But I firmly believe that there's no reason OCD has to hold you back from getting what you want out of life.

Effective treatment can turn the odds in your favor. For most people, OCD is a long-term condition with symptoms that wax and wane, but may never completely disappear. About 85% of people with OCD get better or stay the same over time rather than getting worse. CBT, with or without medication, greatly improves your chances of being among those who actually improve. And sticking to your treatment plan for as long as recommended helps ensure that the improvements are lasting.

That doesn't mean you'll never have setbacks. It's possible some symptoms might come back, especially during times of stress. The good news is that you'll know right away what the symptoms mean and where to look for help. Don't be embarrassed about returning to your treatment provider for an occasional tune-up. It's not a sign that you've done anything wrong. To the contrary, it's a sign that you're doing something very right, by taking charge of the situation and getting help before the symptoms become severe.

Plan on having lapses, and have your battle plan ready. That way, you may be able keep a short-lived lapse from turning into a full-blown relapse—a return to the old way of being for an extended period of time. And don't be discouraged. It's a lot easier to build on progress you've already made than it was to overcome your symptoms in the first place.

> *Plan on having lapses, and have your battle plan ready.*

What's the Least I Need to Know?

Having OCD alone is difficult enough. Having OCD plus one or more other disorders can seem ridiculously unfair. Yet every time you confront and best your personal demons, you become a braver, stronger person. You might feel scared, confused, and troubled at times, but you'll also have many opportunities to grow.

I wish I could tell you there are easy answers, but there aren't. Overcoming OCD and any problems that go along with it will take sweat and perseverance, but I have confidence you'll be up to the challenge. As time passes, you'll be able to look back and smile at how much you've achieved. I can tell you that nothing is sweeter than the satisfaction that comes from staring down your demons.

Chapter Six

Where I Was Is Not Where I Am

In college, I enrolled in a class called The Therapeutic Uses of Writing—an interesting and somewhat unorthodox class in which psychology and creative writing were intertwined. As students, we were encouraged to keep journals and write about what was bothering us whenever we could. I found myself having increasing difficulty when I would read or write certain words and phrases. They would trigger anxiety and obsessions, which, in turn, would trigger the compulsion to put down what I was working on. Needless to say, this made it hard to get much writing done.

Eventually, it got bad enough that I started e-mailing my writing professors everything I had written so far, even if it wasn't yet complete. When I finally finished a writing assignment, I would e-mail it off right after I typed the last word of the last sentence, sometimes even without spellchecking. The idea was that, even if the next thing I did was to delete my work, I wouldn't lose the bulk of the writing. I could pick up where I had left off simply by contacting my professors and asking them to e-mail me the last file I had sent them.

I should point out that my professors were extremely understanding. Curry College, from which I eventually graduated with a bachelor's degree in creative writing, is known in the educational community for its innovative approach to personal learning styles. I took the initiative in making this work to my advantage, however, and that's what counts. By meeting with the head of the writing department, with whom I would become (and remain to this day) very close, I was able to establish a system for electronically preserving the things I wrote.

When an issue with anxiety-provoking words came up, I started using boldface to highlight the words that bothered me when I sent them to the head of the therapeutic writing course. I began to catalog these words and phrases in a file in my e-mail inbox, eventually creating a spreadsheet of them.

I brought the list of words to Dr. C.'s office, where I exposed myself to the words repeatedly during EX/RP therapy. The goal was to desensitize myself to the words and reduce their anxiety-provoking capability. At the same time, I started composing manuscripts for my therapeutic writing class that contained as many of the words as possible, giving myself further exposure to the words as well as a chance to explore them in class. Gradually, the words came to have less power over me.

Romancing the Illness

My life has been, in a word, interesting—or at least, I like to think so. I've often thought that I would be a drastically less interesting person if I didn't have OCD and hadn't been introduced to this other world of the mind. OCD has touched nearly every facet of my life, and romantic relationships are certainly no exception.

Dating is a horrifyingly wonderful amalgam of ecstatic highs and desperate lows. You learn to interact with someone you're attracted to and to take emotional risks. The search for another person who complements and completes you is one way to learn more about who you are and find meaning in life. That doesn't mean it's always fun, however.

When I speak about OCD at conferences, I'm always surprised by the number of questions I get about my personal life. Teenagers, in particular, want to know about my dating experiences. The first thing I tell teens who say they have trouble dating because of OCD is that *everyone* has trouble dating. Let's face it: Dating can be exhilarating, especially when you find the right person, but it can also be a pretty scary experience.

Telling the other person about my OCD was once one of the more intimidating parts of dating. By now, though, I've gotten so comfortable that I hardly realize I'm doing it until I hear the word "obsession" come out of my mouth. At that point, I'm mid-sentence, and it's a little too late to assess whether or not this was a good time to dive into the subject. But my philosophy is simple: If I've been hanging out with someone for a few weeks and she hasn't already noticed that I have OCD—or at least, that something OCD-like is going on with me, even if she doesn't know what to call it yet—then she isn't very observant. And that's not a good sign, since I like girls who are smart, attentive, and engaging.

This is not to say that my opener when I first meet someone is, "Hello. My name is Jared, and I have obsessive-compulsive disorder." The key is letting this information out of the bag when the time seems natural. That's what I did when I met a girl through the radio station where I worked. She was amazing and fit all the criteria I mentioned in the previous paragraph. Plus, she was smoking hot and sweet.

I was working in the station's promotions department, putting together flyers and prize packages for listeners. This girl had to complete a certain number of office hours at the station, too, as part of her college program. One evening, she came into my office, and I offered her the task of helping me weed through public service announcements. I had reams of paper all over the office. We were sifting through some of the stacks, looking for ads that would be suitable to put on the air at a nonprofit station.

As we worked, I turned to the girl and asked how she was doing. She gave me a noncommittal answer, to which I replied that I was more than happy to listen if there was something on her mind. Thus began a friendship that turned into a romantic relationship that remains a friendship to this day.

During one of our conversations, I decided to unload a little burden of my own, as I was having a very hard time holding it inside that day. It occurred to me that anyone worth knowing wouldn't hold OCD against me. We talked about a lot of things that day, some of which will remain between us, but it did come out that I had OCD and that it was causing a great many problems in my life at the time. It was one of those bite-your-tongue-and-hope-for-the-best moments.

> It occurred to me that anyone worth knowing wouldn't hold OCD against me.

Her response was curiosity. This turned into a sort of question-and-answer session about OCD. There were a few of those awkward "I do that, too" moments—as it turns out, everyone wants to share what they think of as their obsessions or compulsions. (It's something you'll probably run into and be confused by, too.) But all in all, it was a very good talk.

In a healthy relationship, both people are always learning more about each other. That's one way you know that you're headed in the right direction. People who are true friends may be curious about OCD when they learn that you have it, but they won't hold it against you or think it defines all that you are. It will be just one of many facts they learn as they get to know you better.

Does That Sound Rational?

I have dated people with OCD as well. This isn't the most romantic thing two people can share, but it's also not something you can rule out as a potential bond. My best advice is to make sure you don't feed off each other's symptoms and enable each other's rituals. This is a lot harder than it sounds. It so happens that, as I write this chapter, I'm in a relationship with another OCD veteran.

Without her help, I'm not sure this book would ever have made it from my chicken-scratches-on-paper to my word processor. I'll be forever grateful to Megan for that. Megan helped me to confront my fears about putting my life down on paper, and slowly but surely, I belted out the first chapter with her sitting on the couch near me, watching me sweat bullets. As soon as I hit the last keystroke of the chapter, I heard her voice beside me saying, "Now save it." I didn't have time to obsess over what I had written before we pushed the first chapter onto the Internet and e-mailed it to my coauthor. If you want to know when you've found a really special girl, try having a panic attack around her and see what happens. I had one right after sending off that first chapter, and Megan was there to help me through it.

As I'm writing this final chapter months later, our relationship has evolved and become even closer. From time to time, when I'm in the middle of explaining whatever I'm anxious about, Megan will stop me short by asking, "Does that sound rational to you?" Confronted by this question, I usually have to admit that my fears have no rational premise, although it may take a little thought and discussion. Recently, though, when Megan asked that same question, I simply replied, "No, it's not rational, is it?" And that was that. Even Megan remarked at how quickly that particular episode was put to rest. What can I say? When a girl makes a point, sometimes you just have to concede.

The One-Shower Rule

It was also Megan who helped me develop the One-Shower Rule for keeping my washing rituals in check. It all started one day in winter, when I found myself feeling distracted and distressed after school. Back in my dorm room, depressed and a little beaten, I undressed, pulled my towel off the peg on the back of my door, and locked myself in the bathroom. Nine showers later, I was in tears. Looking back, I'm not sure exactly what obsessive train of thought set off the compulsive washing, but I do know that my anxiety had a mighty grip on me that day.

Still in my towel, sitting otherwise naked on the floor of my room, I called one of my closest friends on campus and broke down on the phone, explaining everything. In many ways, it was reminiscent of the time I broke down in the locker room during junior high. Both occurrences forced me to admit to myself that I was not nearly as much in control of my situation as I wanted to believe.

That night, I recounted the day's events to Megan, who listened carefully and attentively as always. When I was done telling my tale of OCD woe, she asked me if there was anything she could do to help. After a few minutes' thought, I took her up on her offer and laid out some ground rules for myself: Under no circumstances was I to take more than one shower a day, I told Megan. Just to make sure there were no ambiguities, I defined a single shower as the activity from the time the water started running to the time it was turned off. After the knob was turned and the water stopped running, that shower was over. Furthermore, I was not allowed to turn the water back on, even to watch from the dry bathroom. Megan would be my support person, reminding me of the rules when I needed a nudge in the right direction.

At first, I'll admit, my plan yielded a lot of communications yelled through the bathroom door that sounded something like, "*I can hear the water running again, Jared!*" Within two weeks, however, I had managed to control my urge to play with the shower controls. If I didn't finish shaving in the one shower I was allotted, I would emerge with half a beard, but I still stuck to the One-Shower Rule.

This type of rule isn't restricted to showers, either. If you find yourself doing anything for reasons that are clearly obsessive-compulsive, you can put a limit on the activity. For instance, if you brush your teeth excessively, you can set a limit on the amount of time allotted for tooth brushing each day. To make this work, I recommend finding your own Megan—someone you know and trust who can help you stick to your plan. Give your support person permission to remind you of your vow; for example, to only brush your teeth three times a day for five to ten minutes at a time. Once given, this type of permission needs to be irrevocable. Since it can't be taken back, be sure you think it through first and know what you're getting into.

Sweet Stink of Success

When you spend your whole life staring down dark fears and dangerous invisible and intangible consequences, you see the world differently. OCD helped shape my worldview and make me the person I am today, so perhaps a little ambivalence is natural. On one hand, I desperately wanted to be free of my symptoms. On the other, I was afraid of what would happen after I was liberated.

Finding out that I had OCD was not exactly good news. But once I had accepted the diagnosis and subsequent ramifications, I started to question what my life would have been like if it weren't for the disorder. Easier, no doubt, but also less rich and rewarding in many ways. I believe that having OCD has made me a stronger and more compassionate person, and it has certainly kept me on my toes.

> I believe that having OCD has made me a stronger and more compassionate person . . .

So what can you expect after you start to heal? One of the biggest changes may be having more free time on your hands once rituals aren't eating up hours of each day. My personal advice is to look for a hobby to fill the void—something productive that interests you and challenges you the way OCD did at its worst. This keeps you strong, alert, and prepared to handle the occasional relapse.

I'm an avid martial artist. I currently study Chinese martial arts, but I have done everything from karate and jujitsu to Greco-Roman wrestling. This is one area of my life where it's okay for things not to be perfect. For instance, I'm forced to use other peoples' ratty gloves when I do muay tai kickboxing. You don't know what a horrid stench is until you've smelled your hands after a fight wearing a pair of these gloves. The odor of your own sweat is mingled with that of several years' worth of strangers.' At first, I couldn't use the gloves. My OCD would come on strong, and I would start to panic. Now, however, the odor reminds me that I'm allowed to put obsessive thoughts, compulsive behaviors, and panicky feelings aside. It turns out that success doesn't smell sweet, after all. It smells like old, sweat-soaked leather.

Tooling Up for the Future

There is no miracle cure for OCD, at least not yet. Be patient. Some of the best and brightest scientists in the country are searching for a cure right now. In the meantime, aim to cohabitate with the disease. Just don't be a pushover. During treatment, you'll learn how to show OCD who's really the boss.

It's the job of your therapist or doctor to provide you with tools to fight the thoughts and urges that come with OCD, but it's your job to put the tools to good use. Be prepared to do some periodic upkeep, too. When I was in college, I was under a lot of stress, and my OCD resurfaced hardcore. I beat myself up about it pretty badly at the time, telling myself that it was my fault and I had somehow failed. That wasn't true, though. Managing OCD is a lifelong journey. You may trip and fall occasionally, but you can get back up, brush off the dust, and march on. Each time, you have a chance to learn something new. For instance, you might learn how to solve problems, deal with stressful situations, or persist in the face of obstacles.

You are not traveling this road alone. One of the most important things I've learned is how to ask for and accept help when I need it. This isn't a sign of weakness. To the contrary, it's a sign that I have grown enough to recognize what I can and cannot handle. Some of the best decisions I've ever made involved admitting

Some of the best decisions I've ever made involved admitting that I needed help.

that I needed help. With the tools provided by your treatment providers, you can fight your darkest thoughts and vanquish your most powerful compulsions.

Take back your life. As far as I know—although I could be wrong—you only get one. Then, as you progress, take a moment to look back and smile at how far you've come. I have, and the rewards are sweet. That's why I have written this book.

Frequently Asked Questions

Understanding OCD

Is OCD really a mental illness—and what does that mean anyway?

OCD is considered a mental illness, but that's not as scary as it might sound. A mental illness is a brain disorder that affects your thoughts, moods, emotions, or complex behaviors, such as interacting with other people or planning future activities. Mental illness is a common problem. What's more, the vast majority of people with mental illness are able to function in everyday life, although with some degree of impairment if their symptoms aren't under control.

Okay, I get it, but not everyone is so enlightened. How can I respond when other people make unkind or uninformed remarks?

Stigma refers to stereotyping, prejudice, and discrimination that are directed toward a particular group of people. Unfortunately, there is still a lot of stigma attached to being a person with mental illness. Some people think all you have to do to get better is "pull yourself together" and "stop obsessing," while others regard compulsive rituals as signs of willfulness or stubbornness. You can do your part to battle stigma by politely setting the record straight. Explain that OCD is a disease that is not just in your mind, but also in your brain at a biological level. Although you can't simply will it away, you *can* get treatment. Even the best treatment takes some time to work, though. Let people know you're getting better as fast as you can, and ask for their patience and support in the meantime.

I'm embarrassed to tell my therapist about my obsessions because they seem so weird. How do I know if my obsessions are abnormal even by OCD standards?

When I speak publicly about OCD, I often ask kids in the audience if they can one up me with the absurdity of their obsessive thoughts. I have yet to lose this challenge, although I'm taken up on it every time. The point is that your therapist has undoubtedly heard things that are just as weird, if not weirder. Sharing the thoughts won't cause shock or offense. On the other hand, *not* sharing the thoughts means you may not get the maximum benefit from therapy, since your therapist can't help you work on obsessions that he or she doesn't know about.

By definition, obsessions are upsetting, and some also are quite bizarre. That doesn't make them any more serious than less bizarre ones, however. In fact, virtually everyone, with or without OCD, has weird thoughts on a regular basis. The real issue is how intrusive the thoughts are, how much anxiety or distress they cause, and whether you try to neutralize them with compulsive acts.

Coping at Home

My parents complain about always having to reassure me that things are okay. Why does it bother them so much?

It's annoying to have to say the same thing over and over. But more than that, your parents probably understand that they aren't doing you any favors. Their well-meaning reassurance may actually be helping to perpetuate some of your OCD behaviors. Here's how it works: You have an obsessive thought that leads to a quick jolt of anxiety, followed by the intense need for relief. One way to relieve the anxiety is by asking a trusted authority figure for reassurance: "What if I catch a deadly disease from the other kids at school?" "What if the food is contaminated?" "What if someone leaves the stove on and the house catches on fire?"

Seeing how upset you are, it's natural for your parents to want to quell your anxiety by reassuring you that all is well. The problem is that the reassurance often must be repeated over and over before it neutralizes your obsessive thought and eases your anxiety. And even then, the relief is only temporary. The same scenario may be played out again and again as the obsessive thoughts keep coming back. It becomes not only a repeated pattern for you, but also a habit for your parents that makes the cycle of anxiety and reassurance difficult to break.

Seeking reassurance is a useful way of handling some situations. It can easily get out of hand when you have OCD, though. The good news is that this pattern of behavior can be addressed with CBT. In therapy, you and your parents can learn how to break out of the destructive cycle. Strategies that might help include writing down the reassuring answer yourself rather than asking someone else for it and setting limits on how often you let yourself ask a particular question each day.

My brother and sister give me such a hard time. Why aren't they more sympathetic?

Being the brother or sister of someone with OCD can lead to some complicated feelings. In addition to loving you and caring about your well-being, your siblings may be resentful of all the extra attention you receive. Some also may feel confused about what's happening, guilty because they aren't the ones suffering, worried that the disease will also strike them, embarrassed because your behavior is so "different," or frustrated about having to deal with your compulsive demands.

That's a pretty complex mix of emotions, and it's not uncommon for siblings to feel a bit overwhelmed now and then. Try not to take it personally. Most of the time, they're not unsympathetic, just unable to cope with their feelings. Remember that they're struggling with their own growing pains, too. If the problem continues, call a family meeting to discuss the situation. Also, ask your therapist whether including your parents and siblings in a few sessions might be helpful.

I want the day to get off to a just-right start, but I spend so much time on rituals that I'm often late for school. What can I do?

Get as many decisions as possible out of the way the night before. Lay out your clothes, pack your book bag, and make your lunch. If you need to have a permission slip signed, find resources for a class project, or make arrangements for a ride home, do that the previous night as well. Then set appropriate limits for the tasks that are left. For instance, you might use a timer to control how long you stay in the shower or put a limit on the number of times you let yourself check to see if your homework is in your bag. It also may help to have a support person—for instance, a parent—who reminds you about the limits you've set for yourself.

Getting Treatment

I'm not comfortable with my cognitive-behavioral therapist. Should I look for a new one?

Ask yourself what is making you uneasy. Is it something the therapist said or did, or is it the direction the therapy is taking? The more you can pin down the source of your discomfort, the better you'll be able to evaluate your feelings. It's important to listen to your instincts, especially if anything about the therapist's manner strikes you as inappropriate. But it's also important not to give up too soon, particularly since cognitive-behavioral therapists are in short supply in many parts of the country.

Chapter 2 discusses some of the professional qualifications to consider when choosing a therapist. Beyond that, you should expect to develop a sense of trust and rapport. Ideally, your therapist should be easy to talk to, open to your questions, and willing to help you identify what's in it for you. But keep in mind that it may take a little time to build your relationship. Some people click with their therapists immediately, but others need a few sessions to get comfortable.

The only cognitive-behavior therapist in my area doesn't have any openings for new patients. What can I do?

Ask to be put on the therapist's waiting list. You or a parent also might want to call the therapist's office occasionally to reaffirm your interest. In the meantime, a therapist with a different orientation may be able to suggest some general coping strategies to help you get by until more specific treatment is available. You might even find that the therapist is interested in taking a course or reading a training manual to learn more about how to use CBT techniques to treat OCD. Or the therapist can consult with an OCD specialist about the best treatment strategies for you.

I don't like taking medicine. Are there any herbal supplements that can help my OCD?

Medications for treating OCD sometimes cause unwanted side effects, so you might wonder whether herbal supplements offer a safer alternative. However, just because a product is "natural" doesn't necessarily mean it is harmless. Any product that is strong enough to help your symptoms is also strong enough to potentially cause side effects. Plus, some herbs interact harmfully with certain prescription medications. In addition, most herbal supplements have not been studied in large, well-controlled clinical trials, so there's no way to know whether they really provide the benefits they claim.

Medications must go through a rigorous approval process by the U.S. Food and Drug Administration (FDA). The same is not true of herbal supplements. In the United States, herbal supplements are regulated as foods, which means they do not have to meet the same standards as drugs for evidence of safety, effectiveness, and what the FDA calls "good manufacturing practices." Some published analyses of herbal products have found differences between what's listed on the label and what's in the bottle, so you might be taking more or less of a substance than you think. A supplement label that says it's "standardized," "certified," or "verified" is no guarantee of high quality, since in the United States, there is no legal definition of these terms as applied to supplements.

The bottom line: It doesn't make sense to use an herbal supplement with unproven benefits *in place of* a proven treatment. If you're interested in trying a supplement *along with* therapy or medication, talk to your doctor first to make sure the treatments are compatible. Don't take a higher dose than what is listed on the product label, and if you develop any side effects, stop taking the supplement and tell your doctor.

Going to College

I'll be leaving for college soon. Should I be worried about how I'll adjust?

Starting college is a big transition for everyone, and having OCD only adds to the challenge. Yet while it may take some extra effort and creativity, I'm proof that it's possible to meet the challenge successfully. One key is sticking to your treatment plan in the new environment. If your symptoms flare up, it's also vital to seek help promptly rather than waiting until the problems are severe.

Unfortunately, that's not always what happens. One recent survey of 2,785 college students found that, of those with significant symptoms of anxiety or depression, more than half did not seek professional help. What makes the findings even more noteworthy is that the survey was done at a large public university where students had access to free mental health and counseling services.

A little advance planning can make a big difference. While you're checking out dorm rooms, courses, and nightlife, ask about what kinds of counseling and mental health services are available on campus. Student counseling centers often provide excellent guidance on typical college issues, such as roommate conflicts, academic pressure, and mild worries or sadness. But for more severe problems such as OCD, you probably will need to see a treatment provider at the campus medical center or off campus. If you'll be going to college outside your hometown, ask your current treatment provider to help you line up a therapist or doctor in the new location, or contact the student counseling center or campus medical center for a referral.

I'm a college student who is struggling with OCD. What are my educational rights while I work on getting my symptoms under control?

Some students with OCD qualify as having a disability under the law. Section 504 of the Rehabilitation Act of 1973 applies to students in college as well as to younger students. Another law that applies to students at all levels is Title II of the Americans with Disabilities Act of 1990. Both of these laws prohibit discrimination on the basis of a disability, which is defined as an impairment that substantially limits one or more major life activities. However, there are some key changes in your educational rights once you graduate from high school.

Section 504 requires school districts to provide a "free appropriate public education" to each young person in their jurisdiction up through high school age. After high school, this requirement no longer applies. But colleges can't deny you admission simply because of a disability, assuming you otherwise meet their standards to get in. Colleges also must provide appropriate academic adjustments to ensure that they don't discriminate on the basis of a disability.

There are limits on the types of adjustments that colleges are required to make, however. Examples of possible adjustments include reducing your course load, substituting one course for another, or allowing extra time for taking tests. To make such arrangements, you'll need to notify the school that you have a disability and go through the school's procedure for requesting an academic adjustment, which can take some time. You'll probably need to provide documentation, such as a report from your treatment provider, to show that you have a disability that's affecting you at school. For more information, contact the U.S. Department of Education's Office for Civil Rights (800-421-3481, www.ed.gov/ocr).

I'm trying to pick my college major, so I've been thinking a lot about my career goals. What's the best type of job for someone with OCD?

Untreated OCD can make it very hard to function at work. It's difficult to accomplish much when you're always in the bathroom washing your hands, busy counting the ceiling tiles, or preoccupied with thoughts of disease and disaster. The potential for problems exists regardless of the career you choose. On the other hand, with treatment, it's possible to gain better control over obsessive thoughts and compulsive rituals so that they don't interfere with your job performance.

One of the best motivators for sticking to your treatment plan is a life goal that means a lot to you. In short, the best job for someone with OCD, like the best job for anyone else, is one you love and are determined to succeed at. It may take hard work and persistence, but there's no reason OCD should keep you from pursuing your dreams.

Glossary

acceptance and commitment therapy (ACT)   An offshoot of cognitive-behavioral therapy that combines acceptance of inner experience and commitment to behavior change with mindfulness.

anorexia nervosa   An eating disorder in which people have an intense fear of gaining weight or becoming fat, even though they are underweight. People with anorexia severely restrict what they eat, often to the point of near-starvation.

antidepressant   A medication used to treat or relieve depression. Antidepressants are widely prescribed for anxiety disorders as well.

anxiety disorder   Any of a group of disorders characterized by excessive fear or worry that lasts a long time or keeps coming back. The symptoms cause distress or interfere with the person's day-to-day activities and social relationships.

body dysmorphic disorder   A disorder in which people become so preoccupied with some imagined defect in their appearance that it causes serious distress or problems in their everyday life.

bulimia nervosa   An eating disorder in which people binge on large amounts of food, then compensate by such means as forced vomiting, misuse of laxatives or diuretics, or excessive exercise.

clinical social worker   A mental health professional who is trained not only in therapy, but also in patient advocacy.

cognitive-behavioral therapy (CBT)   A form of psychotherapy that helps people learn how to identify and change self-defeating thought patterns and maladaptive behaviors.

comorbidity   The coexistence of two or more disorders in the same person.

complex tic   A sudden, repetitive, coordinated pattern of movement in several muscle groups that serves no useful purpose.

compulsion   A repeated act, either behavioral or mental, that a person feels driven to perform in response to an obsession to keep something bad from happening or to reduce the associated distress.

co-payment   The portion of health care costs that a patient with health insurance is required to pay for covered services.

deductible   The amount of health care costs that a patient must pay out of pocket each year before health insurance starts paying.

depression   A disorder that involves being in a low mood or irritable nearly all the time, or losing interest or enjoyment in almost everything.

***Diagnostic and Statistical Manual of Mental Disorders,* Fourth Edition, Text Revision (*DSM-IV-TR*)**   A manual that mental health professionals use for diagnosing all kinds of mental disorders.

exposure and response prevention (EX/RP)   A form of cognitive-behavioral therapy that is used to treat obsessive-compulsive disorder. The "exposure" part involves confronting the situations that lead to obsessing, while the "response prevention" part involves voluntarily refraining from using compulsions to reduce distress during and after these encounters.

family therapy   A form of talk therapy in which several members of a family participate in therapy sessions together.

generalized anxiety disorder   An anxiety disorder characterized by excessive worry over a variety of things that are related to real-life circumstances.

habit reversal training   A group of psychotherapy techniques that help people with tic disorders learn how to replace one tic with another that is more socially acceptable.

hoarding   The excessive collection of items with little or no apparent value.

hospitalization   Inpatient treatment in a facility that provides intensive, specialized care and close, round-the-clock monitoring.

hypochondriasis   A disorder in which people become preoccupied with the idea that they have a serious illness, based on their misinterpretation of harmless body signs and sensations.

imagined exposure   A technique in exposure and response prevention. It involves exposure to an anxiety-provoking situation through mental imagery.

individualized education program (IEP)   A written educational plan for a student who qualifies for services under the Individuals with Disabilities Education Improvement Act of 2004.

Individuals with Disabilities Education Improvement Act of 2004 (IDEA)   A federal law that applies to students who have a disability that impacts their ability to benefit from general educational services.

in vivo exposure   A technique in exposure and response prevention. It involves exposure to an anxiety-provoking situation in the real world.

learning disorder   A condition that adversely affects performance at school or the ability to get along in everyday situations that call for reading, writing, or math.

Medicaid   A government program that provides health insurance to eligible low-income and disabled individuals.

medical necessity   A standard used by many insurance plans in determining whether to pay for a health care service. To satisfy this standard, the service must be deemed medically appropriate and necessary to meet a patient's health care needs.

mental health counselor   A mental health professional who typically combines therapy with problem-solving techniques.

mental illness   A brain disorder that affects your thoughts, moods, emotions, or complex behaviors, such as interacting with other people or planning future activities.

mindfulness   A form of meditation that involves fully focusing attention on whatever is being experienced here and now without judging or reacting to it.

modeling   A technique in exposure and response prevention. The therapist demonstrates coming into contact with an anxiety-provoking situation without resorting to compulsive rituals.

neurotransmitter   A chemical that acts as a messenger within the brain.

obsession   A recurring thought or mental image that seems intrusive and inappropriate, and that causes anxiety and distress.

obsessive-compulsive disorder (OCD)   A mental disorder characterized by recurring, uncontrollable obsessions and compulsions.

obsessive-compulsive personality disorder (OCPD)   A disorder characterized by a preoccupation with control, order, and perfectionism that is long-lasting and seen in a wide range of settings.

obsessive-compulsive spectrum disorder   Any of a group of disorders that resemble obsessions or compulsions and may respond to some of the same treatments as OCD.

panic attack   A sudden, unexpected wave of intense fear and apprehension that is accompanied by physical symptoms, such as a rapid heart rate, shortness of breath, or sweating.

panic disorder   An anxiety disorder characterized by the repeated occurrence and persistent fear of spontaneous panic attacks. The fear stems from the belief that such attacks will result in a catastrophe, such as having a heart attack.

pediatric autoimmune neuropsychiatric disorders associated with streptococcal infections (PANDAS)   An uncommon form of childhood obsessive-compulsive disorder that is brought on by a strep infection.

placebo   A sugar pill that looks like the real medication but doesn't contain an active ingredient.

post-traumatic stress disorder (PTSD)   An anxiety disorder that develops after exposure to a traumatic event. Symptoms include re-experiencing the trauma, avoidance, emotional numbing, and increased arousal.

psychiatric nurse   An advanced practice registered nurse with specialized training in mental health care. Treatment may involve providing therapy or, in many states, prescribing medication.

psychiatrist   A medical doctor who specializes in the diagnosis and treatment of mental illnesses and emotional problems. Treatment usually includes prescribing and monitoring medication.

psychologist   A mental health professional who provides assessment and treatment for mental and emotional disorders. Treatment usually consists of therapy or other psychological techniques.

randomized controlled trial   A study in which participants are randomly assigned to a treatment group or a control group. This study design lets researchers determine which changes in the treatment group over time are due to the treatment itself.

scrupulosity   An excessive concern about offending God, committing a sin, having blasphemous thoughts, or doing something immoral.

Section 504   A section of the Rehabilitation Act of 1973 that applies to students who have a physical or mental impairment that substantially limits one or more major life activity.

selective serotonin reuptake inhibitor (SSRI)   A medication that increases the available supply of serotonin in the brain. Although SSRIs are classified as antidepressants, they're also commonly prescribed for the treatment of OCD and other anxiety disorders.

serotonin   A neurotransmitter that helps regulate mood, sleep, appetite, and sexual drive. Low levels of serotonin have been linked to both anxiety and depression.

serotonin transporter (SERT) gene   A gene that helps regulate serotonin concentrations in the brain. It is a major site of action for selective serotonin reuptake inhibitor (SSRI) medications.

social anxiety disorder   An anxiety disorder characterized by marked fear in social situations that involve being around unfamiliar people or the possibility of scrutiny by others.

specific phobia   An anxiety disorder characterized by an intense fear that is focused on a particular animal, object, activity, or situation, and that is out of proportion to any real threat.

State Child Health Insurance Program (SCHIP)   A government program that provides health insurance for the children in certain lower-income families who aren't eligible for Medicaid.

stigma   Stereotyping, prejudice, and discrimination that are directed toward a particular group of people.

substance abuse   The use of alcohol or other drugs despite negative consequences, such as dangerous behavior while under the influence or substance-related personal, social, or legal problems.

support group   A group of people with a common problem who get together to share emotional support, practical advice, and sometimes educational resources.

tic   A sudden, rapid, repetitive movement or vocalization that serves no useful purpose.

Tourette's syndrome   A disorder characterized by frequent, multiple physical and vocal tics.

trichotillomania   A disorder in which people feel driven to pull out their own hair, leading to noticeable hair loss.

Resources

Organizations

All of these organizations provide information about some aspect of OCD or mental illness. Those marked with an asterisk (*) also offer a toll-free phone number or searchable online directory for locating mental health care providers.

Active Minds on Campus
1875 Connecticut Ave. NW, Suite 418
Washington, DC 20009
(202) 719-1177
www.activemindsoncampus.org

*American Academy of Child and Adolescent Psychiatry
3615 Wisconsin Ave. NW
Washington, DC 20016
(202) 966-7300
www.aacap.org
www.parentsmedguide.org

*American Psychiatric Association
1000 Wilson Blvd., Suite 1825
Arlington, VA 22209
(888) 357-7924
www.psych.org
www.healthyminds.org
www.parentsmedguide.org

*American Psychological Association
750 First St. NE
Washington, DC 20002
(800) 374-2721
www.apa.org
www.apahelpcenter.org
www.psychologymatters.org

*Anxiety Disorders Association of America
8730 Georgia Ave., Suite 600
Silver Spring, MD 20910
(240) 485-1001
www.adaa.org
www.gotanxiety.org

*Association for Behavioral and Cognitive Therapies
305 Seventh Ave., 16th Floor
New York, NY 10001
(212) 647-1890
www.abct.org

Bazelon Center for Mental Health Law
1101 15th St. NW, Suite 1212
Washington, DC 20005
(202) 467-5730
www.bazelon.org

Freedom From Fear
308 Seaview Ave.
Staten Island, NY 10305
(718) 351-1717
www.freedomfromfear.org

Mental Health America
2000 N. Beauregard St., 6th Floor
Alexandria, VA 22311
(800) 969-6642
www.mentalhealthamerica.net

NARSAD, The National Mental Health Research Association
60 Cutter Mill Rd., Suite 404
Great Neck, NY 11021
(800) 829-8289
www.narsad.org

National Alliance on Mental Illness
Colonial Place Three
2107 Wilson Blvd., Suite 300
Arlington, VA 22201
(800) 950-6264
www.nami.org

*National Association of Social Workers
750 First Street NE, Suite 700
Washington, DC 20002
(202) 408-8600
www.socialworkers.org
www.helpstartshere.org

National Institute of Mental Health
6001 Executive Blvd., Room 8184, MSC 9663
Bethesda, MD 20892
(866) 615-6464
www.nimh.nih.gov

*National Mental Health Information Center
P.O. Box 42557
Washington, DC 20015
(800) 789-2647
www.mentalhealth.samhsa.gov

*Obsessive-Compulsive Foundation
676 State St.
New Haven, CT 06511
(203) 401-2070
www.ocfoundation.org

Parent Advocacy Coalition for Educational Rights
8161 Normandale Blvd.
Minneapolis, MN 55437
(952) 838-9000
www.pacer.org

Books
Some of these books are more challenging to read than others, but all are well worth the effort. Those written specifically for teens or young adults are marked with a dagger (†).

Foa, Edna B., and Reid Wilson. *Stop Obsessing! How to Overcome Your Obsessions and Compulsions* (rev. ed.). New York: Bantam, 2001.

†Hyman, Bruce M., and Cherry Pedrick. *Obsessive-Compulsive Disorder.* Minneapolis, MN: Twenty-First Century Books, 2003.

Hyman, Bruce M., and Cherry Pedrick. *The OCD Workbook: Your Guide to Breaking Free From Obsessive-Compulsive Disorder* (2nd ed.). Oakland, CA: New Harbinger, 2005.

Neziroglu, Fugen, Jerome Bubrick, and Jose A. Yaryura-Tobias. *Overcoming Compulsive Hoarding: Why You Save and How You Can Stop.* Oakland, CA: New Harbinger, 2004.

Panzel, Fred. *Obsessive-Compulsive Disorders: A Complete Guide to Getting Well and Staying Well.* New York: Oxford University Press, 2000.

Steketee, Gail, and Randy O. Frost. *Compulsive Hoarding and Acquiring: Workbook.* New York: Oxford University Press, 2007.

Fiction

†Hesser, Terry Spencer. *Kissing Doorknobs.* New York: Laurel Leaf Books, 1998.

†Tashjian, Janet. *Multiple Choice.* New York: Henry Holt, 1999.

Memoirs

Bell, Jeff. *Rewind, Replay, Repeat: A Memoir of Obsessive-Compulsive Disorder.* Center City, MN: Hazelden, 2007.

Colas, Emily. *Just Checking: Scenes From the Life of an Obsessive-Compulsive.* New York: Washington Square Press, 1998.

Deane, Ruth. *Washing My Life Away: Surviving Obsessive-Compulsive Disorder.* Philadelphia: Jessica Kingsley Publishers, 2005.

Summers, Marc, with Eric Hollander. *Everything in Its Place: My Trials and Triumphs With Obsessive Compulsive Disorder.* New York: Tarcher/Putnam, 2000.

Traig, Jennifer. *Devil in the Details: Scenes From an Obsessive Girlhood.* New York: Little, Brown and Company, 2004.

Wilensky, Amy S. *Passing for Normal: A Memoir of Compulsion.* New York: Broadway Books, 1999.

Web Sites

Compulsive Hoarding, Obsessive-Compulsive Foundation,
    www.ocfoundation.org/hoarding

MindZone, Annenberg Foundation Trust at Sunnylands with the Annenberg Public Policy Center of the University of Pennsylvania, www.CopeCareDeal.org

Obsessive Compulsive Foundation of Metropolitan Chicago, www.ocfchicago.org

Organized Chaos, Obsessive-Compulsive Foundation,
    www.ocfoundation.org/organizedchaos
Pediatric Obsessive Compulsive Disorder Research, National Institute of Mental
    Health, intramural.nimh.nih.gov/pocd
TeensHealth, Nemours Foundation, www.teenshealth.org

Help for Related Problems

Anxiety Disorders

BOOK

Ford, Emily, with Michael R. Liebowitz and Linda Wasmer Andrews. *What You
    Must Think of Me: A Firsthand Account of One Teenager's Experience With Social
    Anxiety Disorder.* New York: Oxford University Press with the Annenberg
    Foundation Trust at Sunnylands and the Annenberg Public Policy Center at the
    University of Pennsylvania, 2007.

Body Dysmorphic Disorder

BOOKS

Phillips, Katharine E. *The Broken Mirror: Understanding and Treating Body
    Dysmorphic Disorder* (rev. ed.). New York: Oxford University Press, 2005.
Wilhelm, Sabine. *Feeling Good About the Way You Look: A Program for Overcoming
    Body Image Problems.* New York: Guilford Press, 2006.

Depression

ORGANIZATIONS

Depression and Bipolar Support Alliance, (800) 826-3632, www.dbsalliance.org
Families for Depression Awareness, (781) 890-0220, www.familyaware.org

BOOK

Irwin, Cait, with Dwight L. Evans and Linda Wasmer Andrews. *Monochrome Days:
    A Firsthand Account of One Teenager's Experience With Depression.* New York:
    Oxford University Press with the Annenberg Foundation Trust at Sunnylands
    and the Annenberg Public Policy Center at the University of Pennsylvania,
    2007.

Eating Disorders

ORGANIZATIONS

Academy for Eating Disorders, (847) 498-4274, www.aedweb.org

National Association of Anorexia Nervosa and Associated Disorders, (847) 831-3438, www.anad.org

National Eating Disorders Association, (800) 931-2237, www.nationaleatingdisorders.org

BOOK

Arnold, Carrie, with B. Timothy Walsh. *Next to Nothing: A Firsthand Account of One Teenager's Experience With an Eating Disorder.* New York: Oxford University Press with the Annenberg Foundation Trust at Sunnylands and the Annenberg Public Policy Center at the University of Pennsylvania, 2007.

WEB SITE

Anorexia Nervosa and Related Eating Disorders, www.anred.com

Learning Disorders

ORGANIZATIONS

International Dyslexia Association, (410) 296-0232, www.interdys.org

National Center for Learning Disabilities, (888) 575-7373, www.ncld.org

WEBSITE

LD OnLine, www.ldonline.org

Substance Abuse

ORGANIZATIONS

Alcoholics Anonymous, (212) 870-3400 (check your phone book for a local number), www.aa.org

American Council for Drug Education, (800) 488-3784, www.acde.org

Narcotics Anonymous, (818) 773-9999, www.na.org

National Council on Alcoholism and Drug Dependence, (800) 622-2255, www.ncadd.org

National Institute on Alcohol Abuse and Alcoholism, (301) 443-3860, www.niaaa.nih.gov, www.collegedrinkingprevention.gov, www.thecoolspot.gov

National Institute on Drug Abuse, (301) 443-1124, www.drugabuse.gov,
www.inhalants.drugabuse.gov, www.teens.drugabuse.gov, www.clubdrugs.gov,
www.marijuana-info.org

Partnership for a Drug-Free America, (212) 922-1560, www.drugfree.org,
www.checkyourself.com

Substance Abuse and Mental Health Services Administration, (800) 729-6686,
www.ncadi.samhsa.gov, www.csat.samhsa.gov, www.prevention.samhsa.gov

BOOK

Keegan, Kyle, with Howard B. Moss. *Chasing the High: A Firsthand Account of One Young Person's Experience With Substance Abuse.* New York: Oxford University Press with the Annenberg Foundation Trust at Sunnylands and the Annenberg Public Policy Center at the University of Pennsylvania, 2008.

WEB SITES

Facts on Tap, Phoenix House, www.factsontap.org

Freevibe, National Youth Anti-Drug Media Campaign, www.freevibe.com

Suicidal Thoughts

ORGANIZATIONS

American Foundation for Suicide Prevention, (888) 333-2377, www.afsp.org

Jed Foundation, (212) 647-7544, www.jedfoundation.org

Suicide Awareness Voices of Education, (952) 946-7998, www.save.org

Suicide Prevention Action Network USA, (202) 449-3600, www.spanusa.org

HOTLINES

National Hopeline Network, (800) 784-2433, www.hopeline.com

National Suicide Prevention Lifeline, (800) 273-8255,
www.suicidepreventionlifeline.org

BOOK

Lezine, DeQuincy A., with David Brent. *Eight Stories Up: An Adolescent Chooses Hope Over Suicide.* New York: Oxford University Press with the Annenberg Foundation Trust at Sunnylands and the Annenberg Public Policy Center at the University of Pennsylvania, 2008.

Tourette's syndrome

ORGANIZATION

Tourette Syndrome Association, (718) 224-2999, www.tsa-usa.org

WEB SITE

Worldwide Education and Awareness for Movement Disorders, www.wemove.org

Trichotillomania

ORGANIZATION

Trichotillomania Learning Center, (831) 457-1004, www.trich.org

Bibliography

Books

American Psychiatric Association. *Diagnostic and Statistical Manual of Mental Disorders* (4th ed., text revision). Washington, DC: American Psychiatric Association, 2000.

Antony, Martin M., Christine Purdon, and Laura J. Summerfeldt (Eds.). *Psychological Treatment of Obsessive-Compulsive Disorder: Fundamentals and Beyond.* Washington, DC: American Psychological Association, 2007.

Evans, Dwight L., Edna B. Foa, Raquel E. Gur, Herbert Hendin, Charles P. O'Brien, Martin E. P. Seligman, and B. Timothy Walsh (Eds.). *Treating and Preventing Adolescent Mental Health Disorders: What We Know and What We Don't Know.* New York: Oxford University Press with the Annenberg Foundation Trust at Sunnylands and the Annenberg Public Policy Center of the University of Pennsylvania, 2005.

Foa, Edna B., and Linda Wasmer Andrews. *If Your Adolescent Has an Anxiety Disorder: An Essential Resource for Parents.* New York: Oxford University Press with the Annenberg Foundation Trust at Sunnylands and the Annenberg Public Policy Center at the University of Pennsylvania, 2006.

Jenike, Michael A., Lee Baer, and William E. Minichiello. *Obsessive-Compulsive Disorders: Practical Management* (3rd ed.). St. Louis, MO: Mosby, 1998.

March, John S., and Karen Mulle. *OCD in Children and Adolescents: A Cognitive-Behavioral Treatment Manual.* New York: Guilford Press, 1998.

Morris, Tracy L., and John S. March (Eds.). *Anxiety Disorders in Children and Adolescents* (2nd ed.). New York: Guilford Press, 2004.

Ollendick, Thomas H., and John S. March. *Phobic and Anxiety Disorders in Children and Adolescents: A Clinician's Guide to Effective Psychosocial and Pharmacological Interventions.* New York: Oxford University Press, 2004.

Steketee, Gail, and Teresa Pigott. *Obsessive Compulsive Disorder: The Latest Assessment and Treatment Strategies* (3rd ed.). Kansas City, MO: Compact Clinicals, 2006.

Journal Articles

Brown, Richard A., Ana M. Abrantes, David R. Strong, Maria C. Mancebo, Julie Menard, Steven A. Rasmussen et al. A pilot study of moderate-intensity aerobic exercise for obsessive compulsive disorder. *Journal of Nervous and Mental Disease* 195 (2007): 514–520.

Eisenberg, Daniel, Sarah E. Gollust, and Ezra Golberstein. Help-seeking and access to mental health care in a university student population. *Medical Care* 45 (2007): 594–601.

Foa, Edna B., Michael R. Liebowitz, Michael J. Kozak, Sharon Davies, Rafael Campeas, Martin E. Franklin, et al. Randomized, placebo-controlled trial of exposure and ritual prevention, clomipramine, and their combination in the treatment of obsessive-compulsive disorder. *American Journal of Psychiatry* 162 (2005): 151–161.

Hu, Xian-Zhang, Robert H. Lipsky, Guanshan Zhu, Longina A. Akhtar, Julie Taubman, Benjamin D. Greenberg et al. Serotonin transporter promoter gain-of-function genotypes are linked to obsessive-compulsive disorder. *American Journal of Human Genetics* 78 (2006): 815–826.

Kirvan, Christine A., Susan E. Swedo, Lisa A. Snider, and Madeleine W. Cunningham. Antibody-mediated neuronal cell signaling in behavior and movement disorders. *Journal of Neuroimmunology* 179 (2006): 173–179.

March, John S., Martin E. Franklin, Henrietta Leonard, Abbe Garcia, Phoebe Moore, Jennifer Freeman et al. Tics moderate treatment outcome with sertraline but not cognitive-behavior therapy in pediatric obsessive-compulsive disorder. *Biological Psychiatry* 61 (2007): 344–347.

Nakao, Tomohiro, Akiko Nakagawa, Takashi Yoshiura, Eriko Nakatani, Maiko Nabeyama, Chika Yoshizato, et al. Brain activation of patients with obsessive-compulsive disorder during neuropsychological and symptom provocation tasks before and after symptom improvement: A functional magnetic resonance imaging study. *Biological Psychiatry* 57 (2005): 901–910.

Pediatric OCD Treatment Study (POTS) Team. Cognitive-behavior therapy, sertraline, and their combination for children and adolescents with obsessive-compulsive disorder: The pediatric OCD treatment study (POTS) randomized controlled trial. *JAMA* 292 (2004): 1969–1976.

Sareen, Jitender, Brian J. Cox, Tracie O. Afifi, Ron de Graaf, Gordon J. G. Asmundson, Margreet ten Have, et al. Anxiety disorders and risk for suicidal ideation and suicide attempts: A population-based longitudinal study of adults. *Archives of General Psychiatry* 62 (2005): 1249–1257.

Twohig, Michael P., Steven C. Hayes, and Akihiko Masuda. Increasing willingness to experience obsessions: Acceptance and commitment therapy as a treatment for obsessive-compulsive disorder. *Behavior Therapy* 37 (2006): 3–13.

Multimedia Kit

Obsessive-Compulsive Foundation. *OCD in the Classroom: A Multi-media Program for Parents, Teachers and School Personnel.* New Haven, CT: Obsessive-Compulsive Foundation.

Index